D0717947

THE COLLEGE of West Anglia

LANDBEACH ROAD • MILTON • CAMBRIDGE
TEL: (01223) 860701

NORFOLK COLLEGE LIBRARY

3 8079 00050 850 7

PIG AILMENTS:
RECOGNITION AND TREATMENT

To George Sigsworth, formerly Agricultural Officer,
British Broadcasting Corporation,
with grateful thanks for all his help and
encouragement through many years of
radio and television work.

PIG AILMENTS: RECOGNITION AND TREATMENT

TV Book for Pig Farmers

By
EDDIE STRAITON

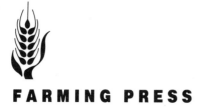

FARMING PRESS

First published 1967
as The TV Vet Book for Pig Farmers.
Sixth edition 1988
retitled:— Pig Ailments: Recognition and Treatment.

Copyright © Farming Press Ltd 1967 and 1988

Reprinted 1991

All rights reserved. No part of this
publication may be reproduced, stored in
a retrieval system, or transmitted, in any
form or by any means, electronic, mechanical,
photocopying, recording or otherwise, without
prior permission of Farming Press Limited.

British Library Cataloguing in Publication Data

Straiton, Eddie, *1917–*
Pig ailments. – 6th ed.
1. Livestock. Pigs. Diseases
I. Title   II. TV Vet. *1917–*. TV Vet book for pig farmers
636.4′0896

ISBN 0–85236–185–8

Published by Farming Press Books
4 Friars Courtyard, 30–32 Princes Street
Ipswich IP1 1RJ, United Kingdom

Distributed in North America
by Diamond Farm Enterprises,
Box 537, Alexandria Bay, NY 13607, USA

Phototypeset by Galleon Photosetting, Ipswich
Printed and bound in Great Britain by
Butler & Tanner Ltd, Frome and London

Contents

GENERAL DISEASES AND AILMENTS

GENERAL HINTS

INDEX

Foreword

By W. T. PRICE, C.B.E., M.C., B.Sc., A.R.I.C.S.

Past Principal of Harper Adams Agricultural College

IT is fortunate that the TV Vet in his third book has dealt with the all-important subject of pigs.

As in his previous publications this well-known author has carried out his original and clear presentation of the subject by a liberal use of some 280 photographs.

Such a pictorial procedure enables the story to be put over in a comprehensive but simple manner which will be clear and helpful to all readers.

In addition to care over the farrowing period, the main theme is that the maintenance of good health is a vital factor in the prevention of disease and how right the author is, for we all know only too well that a sick pig is a "sorry" pig.

Besides the accent on health maintenance there is for each of the diseases and ailments common to the pig, a description of the early symptoms which will lead to a correct diagnosis and prompt liaison between the farmer and the veterinary surgeon. Future success in disease control will depend entirely on a close co-operation between these two.

Although most people fortunate enough to deal in pigs develop an affection for them, nonetheless, the pigs are kept mainly for the purpose of making a profit. This book will certainly help every pig farmer to do just that.

Everyone concerned in the industry and all agricultural and veterinary students should obtain a copy of this informative, useful and practical work for reading, *study* and permanent prominence in their reference library.

Newport,   W. T. PRICE
Shropshire

Author's Preface

THIS is a pictorial representation of the up-to-the-minute disease picture in the pig world expressed in simple, easily-understood terms, with the accent on preventative medicine.

A great deal of research is still going on and no doubt fresh discoveries will be made in the near future. I hope so because there is still a great deal to learn and understand.

No attempt has been made to deal comprehensively with housing, feeding and general management because detailed publications are already available on these subjects. Nonetheless, effective disease control is not possible without a combination of first-class husbandry and the closest co-operation with the veterinary surgeon. The accent must always be on keeping the pigs healthy rather than on treating disease.

I say without any hesitation that the greatest hope for the future lies in commonsense preventative medicine.

I acknowledge with grateful thanks the work and publications of the veterinary scientists without reference to which it would not have been possible to present such an up-to-date disease picture.

And again I express my thanks to my photographers, Mr George Pringle and Mr Tony Boydon, who are responsible for all except three of the pictures.

I should like also to thank the farmers who co-operated in the taking of the pictures, especially Mr Ethan Buxton of Home Farm, Teddesley, Penkridge—the best all-round farmer I know.

Photo Acknowledgments

Oesophagostomum. Taken from Plate 3, Fig. 2 of *Veterinary Parasitology*, 2nd edition 1968, by Geoffrey Lapage, M.D., M.Sc., M.A., F.Inst.Biol. Photograph by G. H. Werts. Published by Oliver and Boyd, Edinburgh.

Ascaris. Taken from Plate 8 of *Veterinary Parasitology*, 2nd edition 1968, by Geoffrey Lapage, M.D., M.Sc., M.A., F.Inst.Biol. Photograph by G. H. Werts Published by Oliver and Boyd, Edinburgh.

Demodex. Taken from Fig. 402 of *Veterinary Parasitology*, 2nd edition 1968, by Geoffrey Lapage, M.D., M.Sc., M.A., F.Inst.Biol. Published by Oliver and Boyd, Edinburgh. Original taken from *Mites Injurious to Domestic Animals*, 1922 by S. Hirst.

GENERAL ADVICE

Advice to Beginners

IN PIG FARMING, time and again, I've seen initial success followed by frustration and failure. Nearly always there has been a reason—often a simple one.

Because of this I would like to set out a few basic rules for the beginner to follow. By doing so he will avoid many of the pitfalls of pig farming.

Experience is absolutely essential. The newcomer *(photo 1)* must spend at least a year working on a successful pig farm before contemplating one of his own.

With experience under his belt he can then set about putting his houses in order. This does not mean spending a fortune on exotic new buildings. It means

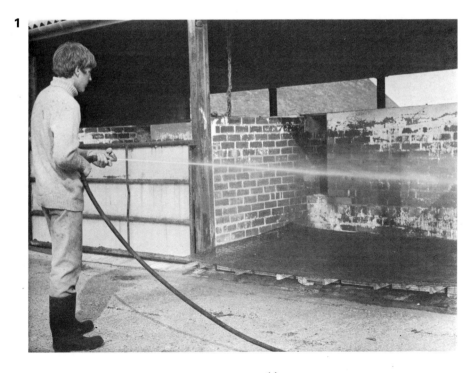

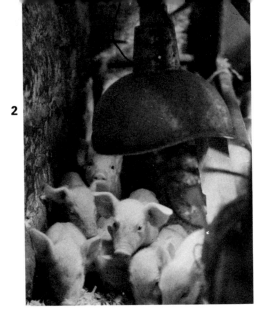

2

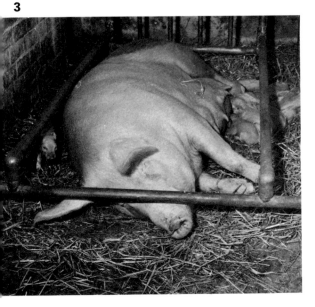

3

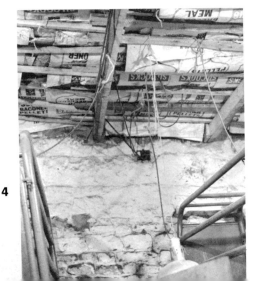

4

an intelligent adaptation of the existing accommodation.

Broadly speaking the sow and piglets require a warm draught-proof pen from which stale air can escape but in which it is possible with the aid of an infra-red lamp *(photo 2)* to keep the creep temperature constant at around 70° F for the first three weeks of the piglets' life.

The floor where the sow lies *(photo 3)* must be insulated so that it provides warmth and dryness. This can be done inexpensively by using farm labour and any one of the many modern insulating materials. Cardboard egg-trays covered over with 1–2 inches of fine concrete will do the job as well as anything.

Draughts can be eliminated by completely closing the pen above and on three sides, i.e. by adopting the kennel system of a house within a house. This can be done in any building simply by providing a false roof *(photo 4)* about three feet above the pigs' backs. The false roof should be removable and made of either wire-netting and straw or wood slats and sacks, but it *must fit tightly* against three closed walls. If there is ample space in front and above the pens then the stale air will escape from under the false roof at a leisurely pace and draughts will not occur. These removable false roofs allow easy cleaning and disinfection.

Using the same techniques the follow-on pens *(photo 5)* should be constructed to provide, by trial and error, a constant temperature of around 60° F with again ample space in front and above the kennels for the stale air to escape. Modern slatted floors are satisfactory and labour-saving.

Water bowls *(photo 6)* correctly sited are absolutely vital. Intelligent use of these simple basic principles can obviate the necessity of considerable capital expenditure in the provision of permanent insulated houses and controlled ventilation. As my friend the late John Cherrington said, 'Folks don't go bankrupt by adapting old buildings—they only go bankrupt when they start building new ones.' Wise words indeed from one of agriculture's most brilliant economists.

Having got the buildings ready the beginner must now make up his mind that never, under any circumstances, will he utilise any building to more than 90 per cent of its capacity. *In other words he must never overstock*. The only way that disease build-up can be avoided is by a rotation of cleaning, disinfecting and resting individual pens *(photo 7)*, and in order to follow this essential routine 10 per cent of the accommodation must always be empty.

Next—the choice of system. I advise the newcomer to pig farming not to attempt for the first year or two at any rate to take the piglets right through from birth to bacon. Instead, he should concentrate either on breeding and selling weaners or in taking the pigs from weaning to pork or bacon *(photo 8)*. Undoubtedly the least disease problem arises with the latter but I suggest that he makes his own mind up after a year or two's experience. If efficient and successful no doubt the birth-to-bacon system will be the natural development. I have found that the pig farmers who sleep the soundest buy at 9 or 10 weeks and sell for pork. In other words they buy after the severe disease period is over and sell again before fresh diseases have a chance to rear their ugly heads.

Next I advise the beginner to utilise to

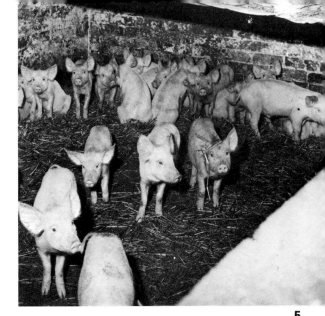

5

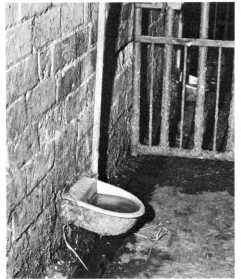

6

7

8

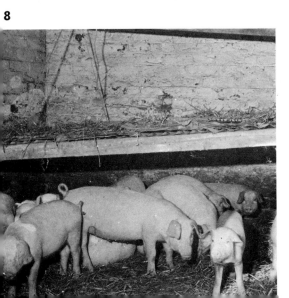

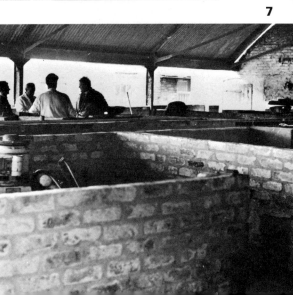

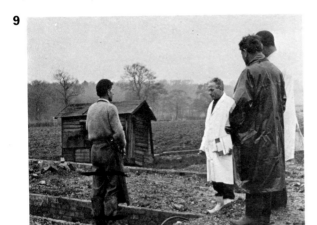

9

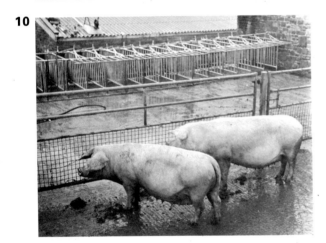

10

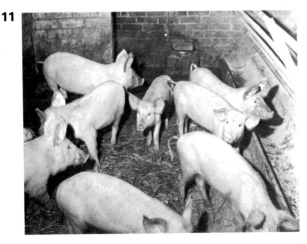

11

the full all available advice, free and otherwise *(photo 9)*. He should draw up a comprehensive feeding plan in consultation with his NAAS adviser or with a reputable feed firm to eliminate all possibility of deficiency diseases and to ensure maximum food conversion rates.

Attachment to the Meat and Livestock Commission is now a must because his future success will depend to a very large extent on careful records and costings. In addition, MLC provides an invaluable up-to-the-minute advisory service.

Also—perhaps the most important job of all—he must commission his veterinary surgeon to draw up a comprehensive plan for disease control. This will include every possible precaution against trouble. In other words, the veterinary surgeon must be given the full responsibility for keeping the pigs healthy. This will probably mean routine inspection visits as well as preventative techniques.

Now, and only now, is the beginner ready to stock his holding *(photo 10)*.

I'd advise him to go all out for hybrid vigour. If breeding, this means purchasing progeny-tested sows of one breed and crossing them with the best possible boar from another breed. Here I'd plump for artificial insemination. The technique can soon be acquired and the potential is tremendous.

If buying stores the best age is 9 to 10 weeks *(photo 11)* and the best source is the small breeder. It will pay handsomely to travel around and contract with the back-door breeders even if it means paying slightly over the odds or a guaranteed price all the year round.

My final word of advice—never must the pig farmer think he knows it all. He will acquire fresh knowledge every day, much of it peculiar but vital to his own enterprise. Let him profit by experience and never hesitate to turn to the specialists for advice.

DISEASES OF THE SOW AND LITTER

1
Farrowing

HEALTH in the pig is of paramount importance because disease costs the British pig industry close on £20 million a year. Three-quarters of that loss occurs either during farrowing or in the five- to eight-week suckling period before weaning.

The process of farrowing *(photo 1)* in the gilt and sow never ceases to amaze me. Through the long protracted labour the mother remains strong, almost unconcerned and fanatically maternal.

Any form of interference at farrowing is not only rarely necessary but it should never—and I mean never—be attempted by anyone other than a skilled veterinary surgeon. The introduction of a hand into the vagina produces an oedema (or dropsy) which retards the whole natural process.

1

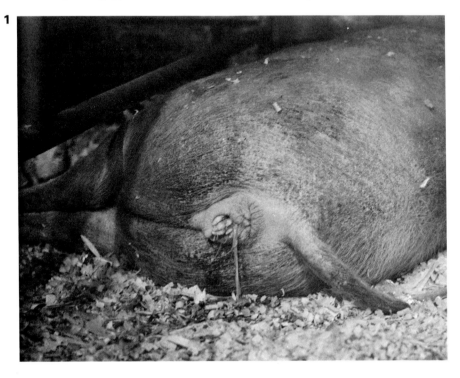

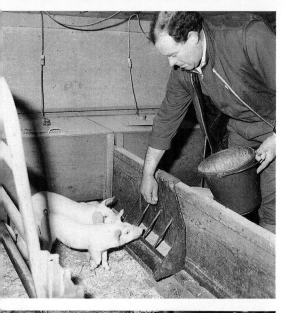

Creep feed (page 12).

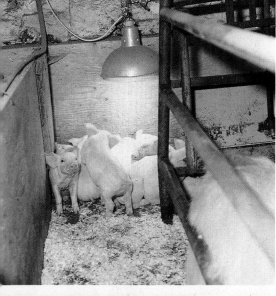

Infra-red lamp to keep creep temperature at around 70°F for the first 3 weeks of the piglet's life (pages 12 and 27).

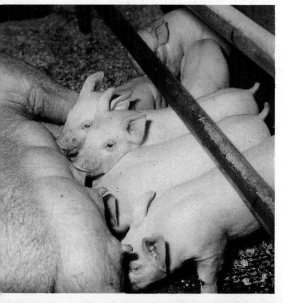

With the advent of high-quality creep feeds many successful pig farmers wean their pigs at 3-4 weeks. This litter is just over a fortnight old.

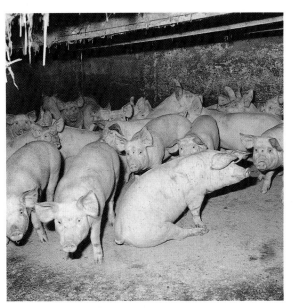

By improvising a kennel within the main house draughts are eliminated. The pen is completely closed on three sides and above by a false roof (page 12).

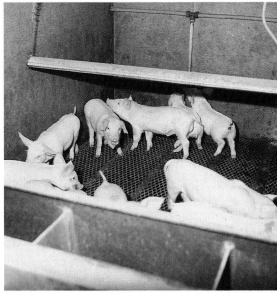

Follow-on pen with highly efficient slatted floors.

The follow-on pens should provide a constant temperature of around 60°F with ample space in front and above the insulated kennels for the stale air to escape.

Controlling the ventilation and temperature in the follow-on pens.

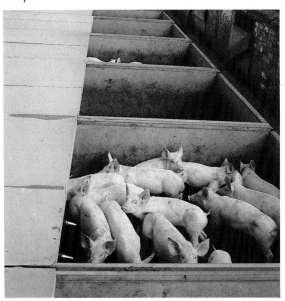

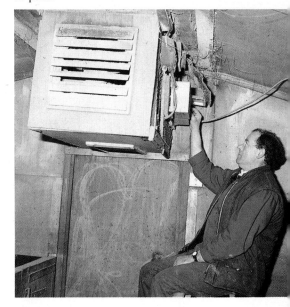

Plenty of time and patience is the key-note to all successful farrowings *(photo 2)*. Occasionally the job may extend over several days, though when this happens it usually means dead piglets. So my advice in all cases of protracted farrowings is to send for your veterinary surgeon. He will probably prescribe daily doses of an antibiotic, but will not introduce his hand unless as a last resort. Just occasionally I have found it necessary to give an old sow a helping hand towards the end of farrowing. But even in these cases, again and again, I have seen the sow complete the job with little effort after she has been given time to regain her strength.

To sum up, therefore, my hints at farrowing *(photo 3)* are: Never panic, have patience and never under any circumstances stick your hand inside. If you think the job is taking too long, send for your veterinary surgeon and let him take over.

Agalactia

This means simply loss of milk or retention of the milk by sows after farrowing. It is caused mostly by mastitis or metritis but can be due to a hormone deficiency usually the milk releasing hormone called oxytocin.

In all cases of agalactia a veterinary surgeon should be consulted immediately.

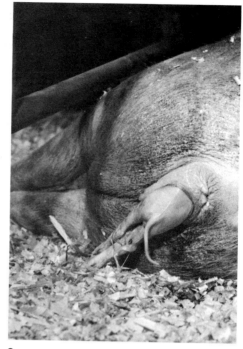

2

3

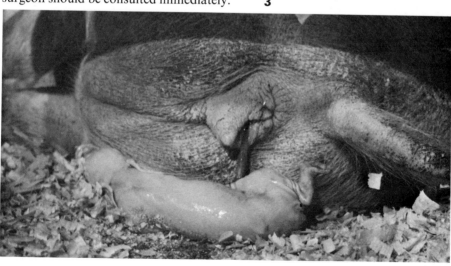

2
Abortion and Stillbirths

IN THE SOW, unlike in the cow and ewe, there are no established specific causes of abortion *(photo 1)*. Nonetheless there are a number of factors which have been shown to be involved. These can be classified as:

1. *Infectious* (caused by bacteria or viruses).
2. *Nutritional and parasitic*.
3. *Mechanical*.

In the infectious type of abortion the organisms shown to have been present are the erysipelas 'bug', the *E. coli* germ, the corynebacteria, a pasteurella, staphylococci, streptococci and a leptospira. The viruses of Aujeszky's disease and swine fever have often been implicated. These bacteria, carried in the

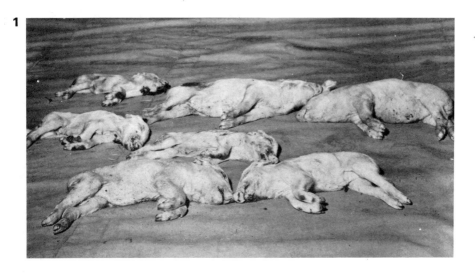

mother's blood, enter the unborn piglets through the navel *(photo 2)* which is attached to the placenta inside the mother's uterus.

Nutritional factors are first of all an obvious lack of vitamin A *(photo 3)*. This can easily happen if, say, a batch of gilts with no access to pasture are fed a home-mixed ration without any vitamin supplement. And, secondly, from ingestion of excess oestrogens from young pastures or plants, or the eating of ergot on barley: also fungi found in mouldy food. Any one of these feed faults can lead to abortions or stillbirths, or both.

Heavy infestation with intestinal parasites can and does cause abortion and certainly is an established factor in infertility.

Mechanical Causes

   (a) Erysipelas vaccination of pregnant animals.
   (b) Bullying or fighting during floor-feeding in a crowded yard *(photo 4)*.
   (c) Travelling.
   (d) Prolonged farrowing.
   (e) Struggling through deep mud.

From my own experience I'd say that wholesale abortion of dead pigs occurs mainly in gilts. Usually, in sows, only part of the litter are affected. I have noticed that the following litters are carried to full term and appear perfectly normal: in other words the gilt or sow doesn't usually abort more than once.

My advice, therefore, in abortion, is to isolate the affected animals for at least a month but not to scrap them. At the same time consult your veterinary surgeon so that he can at least investigate and eliminate any apparent predisposing cause.

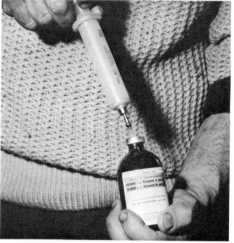

3

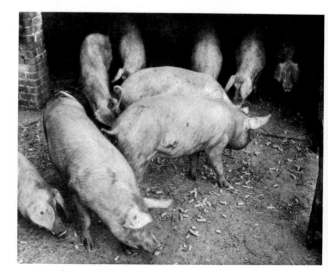

4

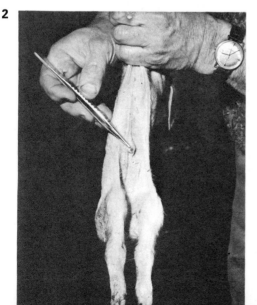

2

Pig Parvovirus

Cause

A small highly resistant virus, the most important and strongest of the group of viruses collectively described as *Smedi*. The pig parvovirus is present in a high percentage of European pigs and manifests itself only when the host's resistance is lowered.

Symptoms

There are no specific individual symptoms so diagnosis of the condition depends on a full knowledge of the herd's history.

What happens is that the virus crosses what we call the placental barrier—that is the membranes which attach the embryo or foetus to the uterus of a gilt or sow—and, depending on when that crossing occurs produces any or all of the following:

(a) Death of the embryos. These embryos are absorbed and lead to:—

(b) Infertility, pseudopregnancy and irregular heat periods.

(c) Mummification of part or of each of the entire litter.

(d) Stillbirths and/or small litters.

At one time abortion was thought to be typical but it is now known that abortion as such is unusual, the tendency being for the gilt or sow to carry the litter to full term or even longer. The virus does not produce clinical symptoms in adult pigs.

Treatment

Must be aimed at prevention.

Prevention

An efficient vaccine called Suvaxyn Parvo 2 (marketed by Duphar of Holland) provides a high degree of immunity in healthy pigs. The dose is 2 ccs given intramuscularly—an initial course of two injections at 3–4 week intervals followed by a booster every 2 years. With gilts and boars the *minimal age for the first inoculation is 5 months*.

As mentioned above the virus is highly resistant against heat and antiseptics, but the most efficient disinfectant is common bleach.

Where vaccine is not available, remnants of mummified foeti and membranes may be 'fed back' to the healthy stock. This is a crude form of management vaccination but it does appear to work.

Smedi

This is the name given to infection by any one of a group of viruses, by far the most important of which is the Parvovirus already dealt with.

Cause

So-called enteroviruses, 4 of which are known as V13, F34, Teschen and Talfan. Teschen disease, a severe form occurs in central Europe and Talfan, a mild disease occurs in Britain.

Symptoms

Teschen: high fever, off food, staggering, followed by stiffness, tremors, convulsions, paralysis and death.

Talfan: affects young unweaned and weaned pigs. High temperature, staggering leading to paralysis or recovery. The affected piglets are often seen in a 'dog-sitting' position.

V13 and F34: may well be responsible for the abortions that were originally blamed on the Parvovirus. They may also contribute to the other reproductive failures already described under Parvovirus.

Prevention

In central Europe a vaccine is available against Teschen but so far no vaccine has been produced against this or the other Smedi viruses that affect British pigs.

Simple Causes of Reproductive Failure

(a) Boar too small.

(b) Failure to serve at correct time.

(c) A low energy diet. See infertility (page 47).

3
Congenital Abnormalities

IT'S IMPORTANT to watch out for congenital abnormalities *(photo 1)* so that the culprit (almost invariably the boar) can be promptly culled.

The congenital abnormalities in order of frequency are:

Hernias or ruptures. These appear either in the scrotum (scrotal hernia) or at the navel (umbilical hernia).

Atresia ani means no open anus for the passage of dung *(photo 2)*. Sometimes, as in this case *(photo 3)*, the piglet is lucky and is able to pass dung through the vulva.

Splay-leg where the hind legs usually splay outwards. The piglet can't get to the teat, is virtually helpless, and is constantly exposed to the danger of death by overlaying. I've noticed that most cases of splay-leg *(photo 4)* seem to occur in Landrace.

Pityriasis rosea. A congenital skin condition, not unlike ringworm. Red eruptions with crater-like edges appear under-

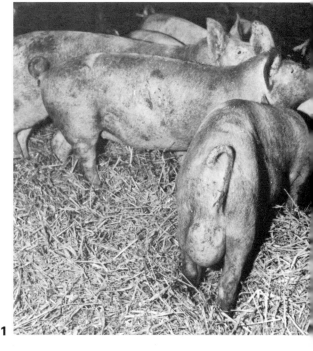

1

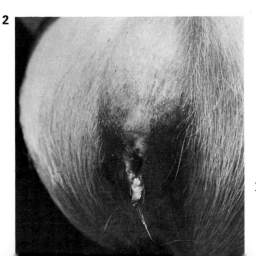

2

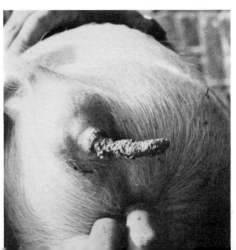

3

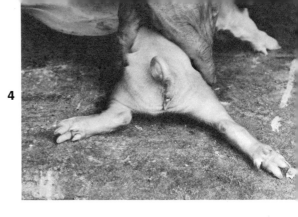

4

neath the belly when the piglets are 3–4 weeks old.

Kinky tail (photo 5) where the piglet's tail has a definite kink in it.

Dermatosis vegetans. A rare condition occurring only in Landrace and Landrace crosses. Worth recording because it is characterised by:

1. A skin eruption at birth.
2. 'Clubbed' or abnormal feet.
3. Death from pneumonia before or shortly after weaning.

Trembling. This can be due to an incipient swine fever infection or to other intra-uterine viruses and bacteria.

When these abnormalities occur the best thing to do is to change the boar immediately and to follow up by carefully testing and recording the new boar on the same sows *(photo 6)*.

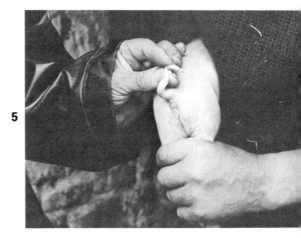

5

So far there is only one apparent congenital abnormality where it is better to cull the sow and that is a condition which we call *Purpura haemorrhagica*. This is characterised by piglets developing, soon after birth, minute haemorrhages in the skin and the mucous membranes of the mouth and nose. On post-mortem examination other minute haemorrhages are found in the internal organs.

If the sow throws one litter thus affected she will continue to do so no matter what boar is used. She should therefore be culled as soon as the condition is diagnosed. But ask your veterinary surgeon to check your diagnosis before getting rid of the sow.

Ruptured pigs can be operated on; splay-leg pigs can be nursed onto their feet; trembling pigs will recover; and a kinky tail makes little difference to performance. But it is wise in all reputable breeding enterprises to go all out to eliminate all these congenital abnormalities by culling.

Less common defects are inverted nipples, cleft palate, one descended testicle (i.e. a crytorchid), thick forelegs, cystic kidneys, legless piglets and barking piglets all of which can be identified by a veterinary surgeon.

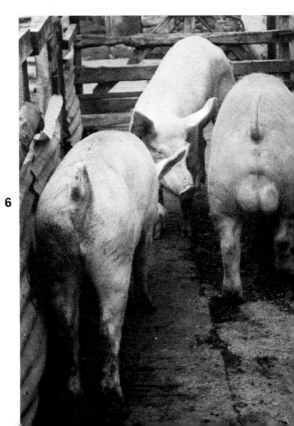

6

4
Milk Fever

I AM often asked if sows can get milk fever *(photo 1)* similar to that occurring in cows. The answer must be 'Yes' because I have seen several cases, though the condition is not by any means common.

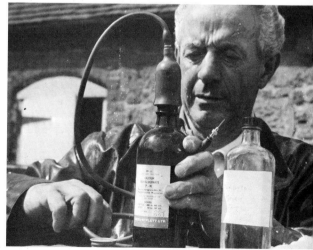

Symptoms

After farrowing, the sow may behave exactly like the cow with milk fever—cold ears, off her food, wobbling about, and then going down and being unable to rise. Her temperature is normal, and she may simply be found down after farrowing. If untreated she will relapse into a coma and die.

Treatment

In the few cases I've seen a spectacular response has followed the subcutaneous injection of a solution of calcium *(photo 2)*. This is definitely a job for the veterinary surgeon because it can be extremely difficult to inject a large quantity of fluid under a pig's skin.

The Thin Sow Syndrome

This is not uncommon and is due to a combination of parasitism, cold draughty housing and inadequate feeding, especially when the sow is suckling the piglets. It can be prevented by sound common-sense management and should be treated along the same lines—namely by maintaining an environmental temperature of 70–72°F, by regular dosing against parasites and by correct feeding *at all times* both during and after pregnancy.

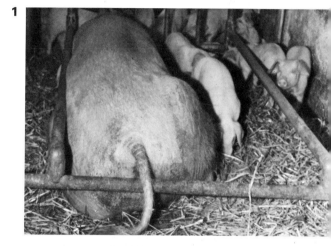

23

5
Mastitis

APART from over-laying, one of the most consistent causes of piglet losses is the lack of milk in the sow. The two most common causes of this milk deficiency are mastitis *(photo 1)* and metritis. In my experience practically all cases of so-called agalactia (loss of milk) in the sow have been due to an incipient (mild) or an acute mastitis.

Cause

The majority of cases of mastitis are caused by the germ *Escherichia coli*. There are 300 dangerous strains of this germ which vary in different parts of the country.

Occasionally, mastitis in the sow is caused by a germ called *Staphylococcus aureus* (which causes black garget in sheep and cattle) or by a germ called *Actinobacillus lignieresi* (also responsible for wooden tongue in cattle). But in sows both the staphylococcus and the actinobacillus cause a more chronic type of infection which often leaves a large hard, ulcerating swelling in one or two quarters *(photo 2)*. Other bacteria are occasionally involved.

Where Does The Germ Come From?

E. coli lives and persists chiefly inside the intestines of many apparently healthy pigs —pigs of all ages, not only sows but weaners and stores. The staphylococcus and actinobacillus usually gain entry

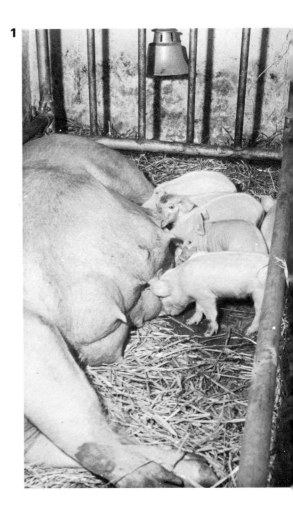

1

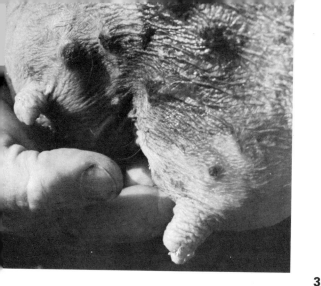

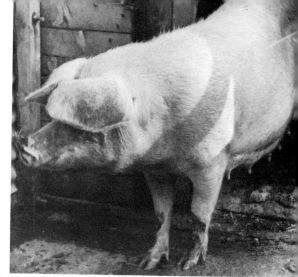

3

through a scratch or a cut *(photo 3)*, though both of them can be normal residents of the udder.

The coli germ which is the most frequent offender causes no trouble whatsoever unless the resistance of the pig is lowered in some way. This lowering of resistance is usually brought about by simple faults in management.

E. coli is passed out in the dung and can live on the pastures for up to two months and inside buildings for approximately one month, but it is important to remember the chief source of *E. coli* is the *pig* itself. At the same time bear in mind that the germs can build up in strength and virulence in continually-occupied pens.

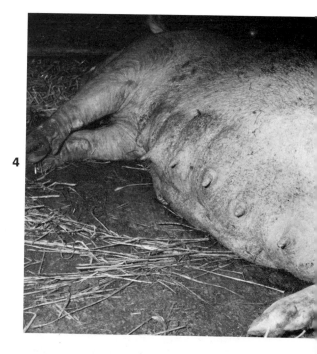

4

Predisposing Factors In Mastitis
Mastitis is often precipitated by a damp dirty floor or a cold draughty farrowing pen *(photo 4)*. It can occasionally flare up as a result of teats being bitten by the baby piglets, or from the irritation of sawdust bedding.

Constipation is another possible predisposing cause.

Symptoms
The first sign is loss of milk *(photo 5)*, and the squealing piglets usually provide the first clue that something is amiss. The sow usually goes off her food and runs a tem-

5

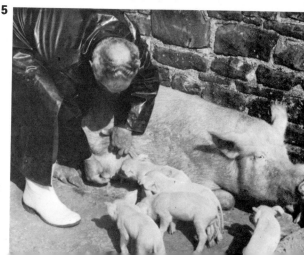

25

6

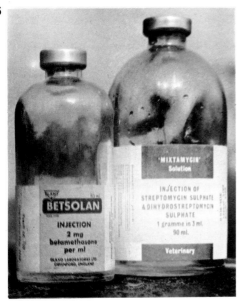

perature of 104°–107°F. She may refuse to suckle her pigs because the udder or part of the udder becomes swollen hard and painful. The milk will be thin, clotty or discoloured.

Treatment

Mastitis usually responds reasonably well to large doses of antibiotic and cortisone given by injection *(photos 6 and 7)* once daily for two or three days. It is very important to spot the condition early and to consult a veterinary surgeon immediately, otherwise litter losses may be heavy. Veterinary supervision is advisable because it may be necessary to type the germ in a laboratory where sensitivity tests can be carried out to find which drug is most effective against it. The odd fatal case is usually complicated by powerful bacteria called klebsiella spp.

Prevention

Obviously it is much better to do everything possible to prevent mastitis. The simple way to do this is to avoid or remove the predisposing factors.

Do not use sawdust bedding; the damp dirty floor can be avoided by insulating with cardboard egg-trays, hollow brick tiles or with any of the other modern insulating materials. If the floor is correctly insulated the straw bedding will virtually powder to dust on the floor surface *(photo 8)*. Where it is not immediately possible or practical to install an insulated floor two preventive injections can be tried.

First of all the sow can be injected with a large dose of antibiotic the day before and the day after farrowing. But never forget that the use of any antibiotic is only a very poor substitute for good management, and correct housing and husbandry must be the ultimate aim.

Secondly, an autogenous vaccine can be used, i.e. a vaccine prepared from the particular coli prevalent on the farm. This is a job for the veterinary surgeon and veterinary laboratory. I have used autogenous vaccines fairly extensively but have found their success variable. Mostly the need for them has disappeared when the other stress factors have been eliminated.

Proprietary vaccines (e.g. Piglet Enteritis Vaccine, Burroughs Wellcome & Co.) are outstandingly successful in some areas, as is the comparatively new

7

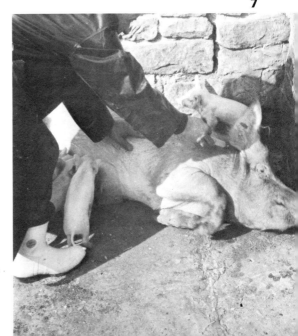

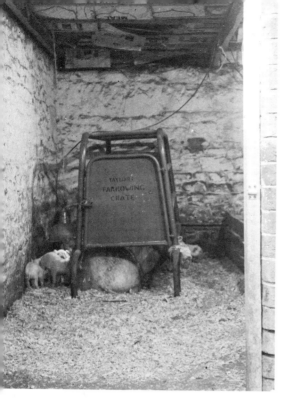

the lamp rises sharply and cold air flows in to take its place, thus producing a dangerous floor-draught. In other words, unless the house is constructed properly an infra-red lamp can do more harm than good.

When building or improvising a farrowing pen for the sow remember this important fact. During farrowing the sow will lose up to 20 degrees of body-heat and unless she is in a place where she can be kept at a comparatively high constant temperature her milk will disappear, the piglets will die and mastitis will be likely to occur.

Constipation—another predisposing cause—can be prevented by isolating the sow 14 days before farrowing and exercising her conscientiously every day. This requires self-discipline on the part of the pigman but the trouble is well worth while. Sensible feeding is also important; the sow should be fed regularly and be given an increasingly laxative diet containing adequate but not excessive protein. A useful

oral vaccine (e.g. Intagen) which is included in certain pig diets.

Such vaccines not only help to prevent mastitis but can also play an important part in controlling all subsequent *E. Coli* infections in the litters.

The sow should be housed in a draught-proof insulated house. It need not be built specially, nor be too elaborate, so long as draught is completely eliminated. Any pig-house can be made suitable simply by making the sow's sleeping quarters compact and completely closed above and on three sides. In the ordinary farm building this can be done simply by providing a false roof approximately 2 feet 6 inches to 3 feet high. Such a roof can be made from wire-netting and straw or wood slats and sacks. It is important, however, that the roof should fit tightly against the three walls to completely preclude the slightest draught.

An infra-red lamp *(photo 9)* is an advantage particularly after the piglets are born. But the lamp loses its effectiveness completely unless a low false roof is provided. In high buildings the hot air around

9

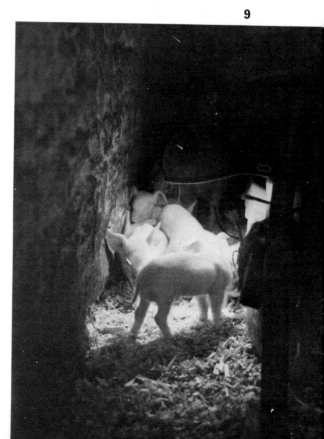

hint is to add liquid paraffin to the meal *(photo 10)*. But perhaps the most important thing of all is to provide an abundant supply of drinking water both before and after farrowing.

To avoid disease build-up (i.e. the germs increasing in strength and virulence within the pens), scrub and disinfect the pen after each litter is weaned and leave completely empty for at least a fortnight. The cleaning *(photo 11)* must be extremely thorough —it's no use playing at it.

Piglets bite the teats only when there are too few teats for the number of piglets or when there is not enough milk. Nonetheless, in all litters, wounds are liable from the sharp, baby incisor teeth. It is wise therefore to clip the teeth of all piglets as soon after birth as possible *(photo 12)*.

A final precaution—wash the sow before putting her in the clean farrowing pen, using the technique advised in the prevention of mange.

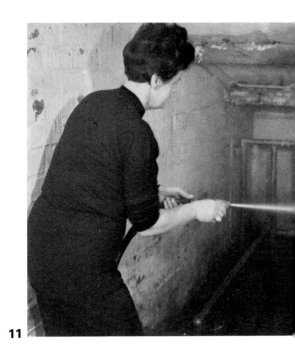

11

10

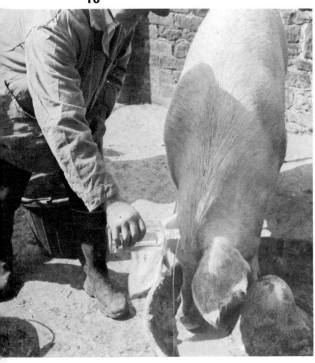

12

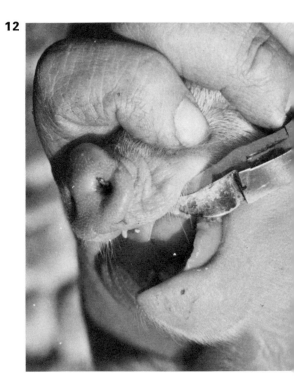

6
Metritis

METRITIS is an inflammation of the uterus or womb of the sow manifested by a nasty discharge after farrowing *(photo 1)*. It causes approximately 30 per cent of sow infertility.

Cause
E. coli. Occasionally other germs are involved especially after the sow has passed dead or putrid piglets. In fact laboratory examination of the discharge may show many other bacteria especially Staphylococci but the trigger factor is usually an *E. coli.*

Where Does The Germ Come From?
Once again the carrier sow.

What Causes It To Flare Up?
In my experience the persistence of metritis appears to depend on the virulence of the coli. While all the management factors are important, the chief one to watch out for

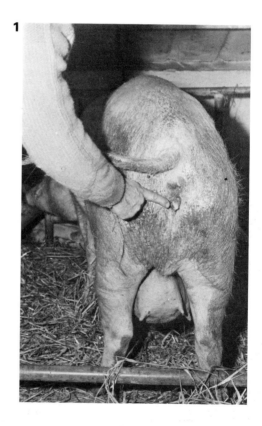

1

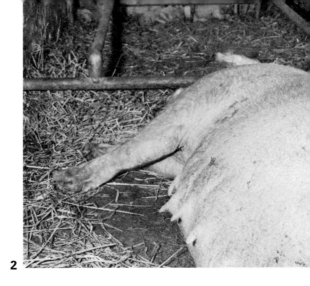

is the disease build-up in farrowing pens which are continually used without rest *(photo 2)*.

Symptoms

The sow may or may not go off her food *(photo 3)* but she is usually sickly and off colour. Her temperature may be normal or raised to 103°–104° F (normal temperature of a pig is 102·5° F). The discharge comprises yellow or dirty yellow pus; it does not usually smell except after the birth of decaying pigs.

Treatment

Metritis, like mastitis, usually responds very well to large doses of specific antibiotics. Two injections on successive days are usually enough, but continual antibiotic therapy produces resistant germs so it's much better to go all out to prevent the disease.

Prevention

Concentrate on reducing the virulence or strength of the *E. coli* by avoiding a disease build-up. To do this it is essential not only to scrub and disinfect *(photo 4)* the farrowing pen after each litter, but to rest each pen completely for at least 14 days before housing the next sow. In addition, eliminate all the other stress factors as outlined in the prevention of mastitis.

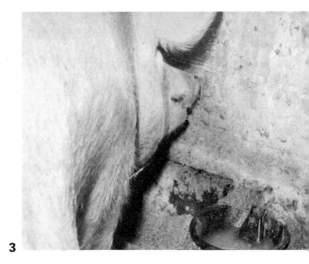

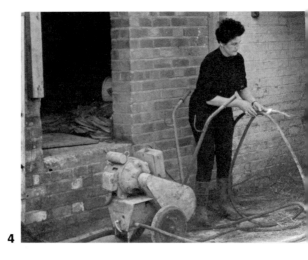

30

7
Baby Piglet Disease

HAVING kept the farrowing sow clear of mastitis and metritis our next breeding hazard is baby piglet disease or scours and deaths in the first few days of life. Baby piglet disease is caused again almost entirely by public enemy number one of all pig breeders—*E. coli*. Just occasionally a bloodstained fatal diarrhoea can be caused by another germ—*Clostridium welchii*—the same germ that causes lamb dysentery in sheep.

Where Does The Germ Come From?
As in the case of mastitis and metritis either from infected pens or from the sows. Most sows act as carriers of *E. coli* and pass the 'bug' on via the dung. This then contaminates the udder and the piglets pick up the germ during suckling. If, of course, the sow has *E. coli* mastitis then the piglets get the germ in the milk *(photo 1)*. If metritis is present the uterine discharge can contaminate the udder.

How Does It Affect The Piglets?
E. coli produces either a septicaemia or a toxaemia (i.e. blood poisoning or contamination of the blood by toxins or waste products excreted by the germ).

1

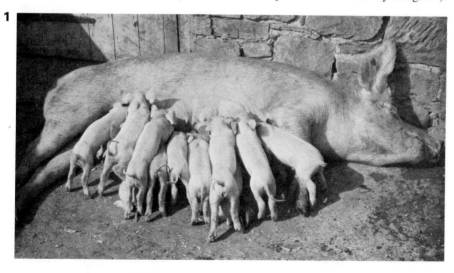

31

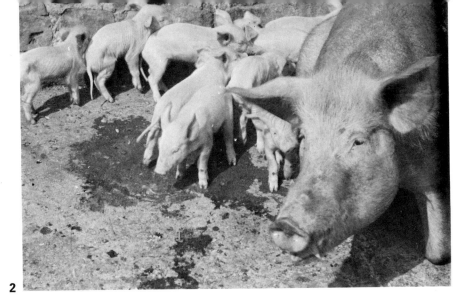

2

Symptoms

Apparently healthy piglets usually about 2 to 3 days old suddenly become dopey *(photo 2)*; their ears become cold and their temperature sub-normal; then they flop about and die within a few hours with or without diarrhoea. This can be treated but it's much better to go all out for *logical control*. In the experience of all veterinary surgeons this type of scour in baby piglets comprises the greatest single source of loss to the pig industry. Thus what I have to say now is probably the most important part of the whole of this book.

The two vital factors in control are:

- To build up the natural resistance of the sow and piglets.
- To reduce the dose of germs to which the sow and piglets have access.

Best way to assist nature by building up the natural resistance of both the mother and litter is as follows:

1. *Keep a closed herd (photo 3).* Remember when strange pigs are introduced they bring different strains of bacteria—also they have to face up to new types of bacteria before they have had a chance to develop antibodies against them.

3

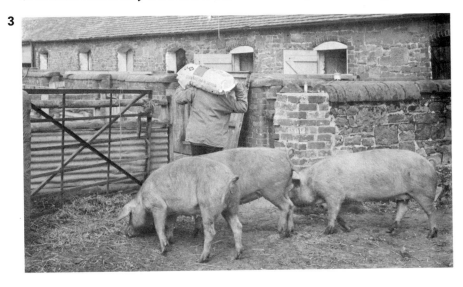

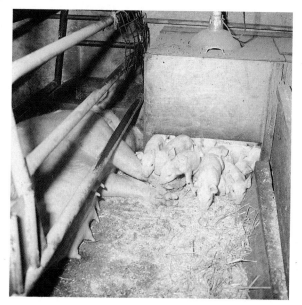

A contented litter at the correct temperature.

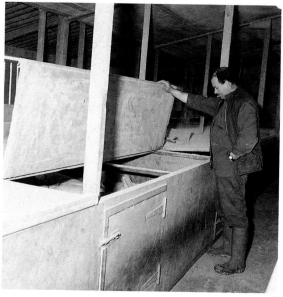

From the follow-on pens to the highly successful solari-type house.

The farrowing pen — insulated, clean and power washed between each farrowing (page 16).

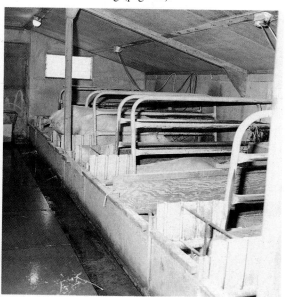

Hernias or ruptures appear at the navel or in the scrotum (scrotal hernia) as below (page 21).

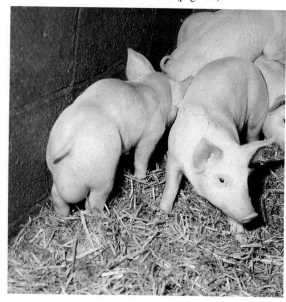

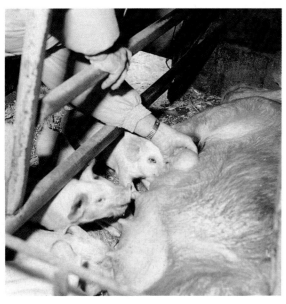

Mastitis in the sow often leaves a large, hard, ulcerating swelling in one quarter (page 24).

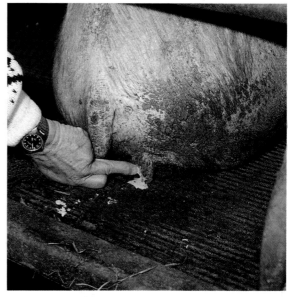

The tell-tale discharge of metritis (page 29).

A damp dirty floor can predispose to mastitis (page 29).

Baby piglet disease, a breeding hazard in the first few days of life (page 31).

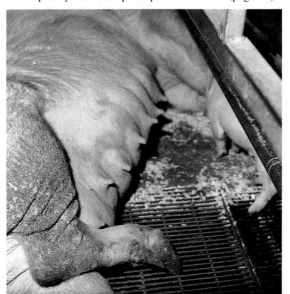

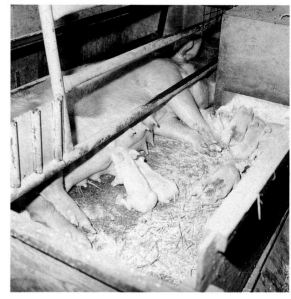

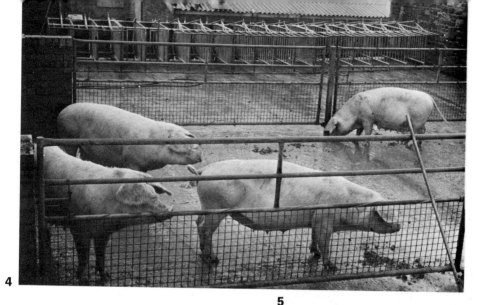

4

5

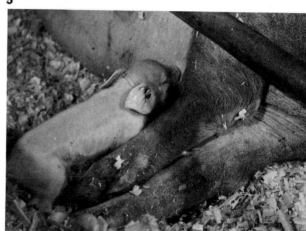

Not only should you try to keep a closed herd, therefore, but for the same reasons you should never under any circumstances be tempted to buy a pregnant sow.

2. If you have to buy the odd replacement, buy it young—about 6 months old —and keep it isolated for at least a month before allowing it to run with the herd.

3. *Mix the gilts with the sows (photo 4)* as early as possible. This gives the gilts a chance to pick up the sows' germs and thus to build up a resistance against these 'bugs' before farrowing takes place. If the gilts can have time to produce antibodies in their blood then these are passed to the piglets in the colostrum, and the scour and deaths are much less likely.

4. *Make sure the piglets get the colostrum or first milk from the sow (photo 5)*. Colostrum contains the essential protective antibodies against scour and is the only certain source for the piglets.

5. *Look after the sow before farrowing* by being careful to avoid constipation. Provide ample exercise *(photo 6)* and wet mashes, and at the same time keep a constant check on her water intake.

6. *Avoid draughts, chilling, or rapid changes in temperature.* Any one of these can lower the resistance of the sow and piglets, and allow the *E. coli* to flare up.

6

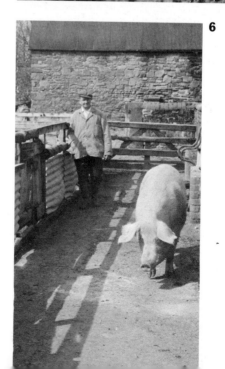

33

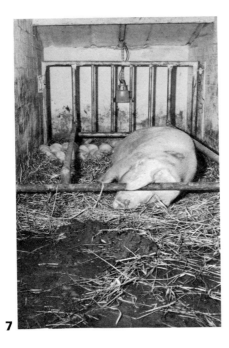
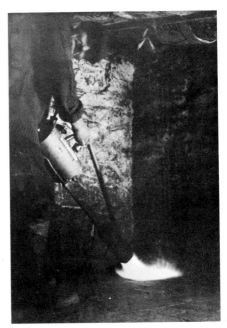

7

8

Keep the creep and pen *(photo 7)* at a constant high temperature of around 70°–75°F.

7. *As a final aid to the build-up of natural resistance vaccinate the piglets, gilts and sows.* Use an enteritis vaccine containing antibodies against your particular strain of *E. coli*. Vaccinate twice—at 6 weeks and again at 2 weeks before each farrowing. Oral vaccines can also be used.

The obvious sensible way to reduce the dose of available germs is by the means I've already described, namely by cleaning, flame-gunning *(photo 8)*, disinfecting, and resting completely for at least a week (preferably a fortnight) each farrowing pen before bringing in the next clean, pregnant sow.

These then are the sensible ways to fight *E. coli* in both the sows and piglets, i.e. by building up natural resistance and by keeping the dose of available germs down to the absolute minimum. If after all this your coli is still so strong that you keep getting odd cases of disease then it is a job for your veterinary surgeon. He will probably type your strain of coli and prescribe a specific antibiotic, but only until such time as your husbandry can be put right and an adequate natural resistance can be fully established.

8

Clostridium Welchii or Enterotoxaemia

(sometimes referred to as Clostridium Perfringens type C)

ENTEROTOXAEMIA is a condition almost identical to dysentery in lambs. It affects baby piglets usually in the first 2 or 3 days of life *(photo 1)*. Fortunately it is not nearly so prevalent as the baby piglet disease caused by *E. coli*: though it occurs much more frequently in Hungary and the USA.

How To Spot Enterotoxaemia

The piglets at one to two days old develop a yellow watery diarrhoea which quickly

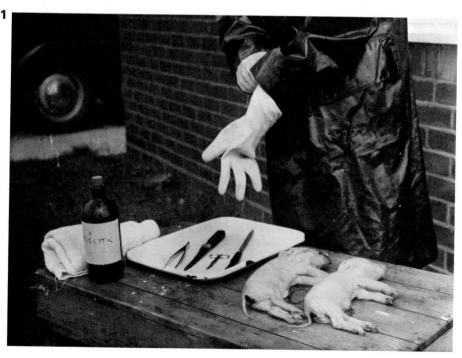

1

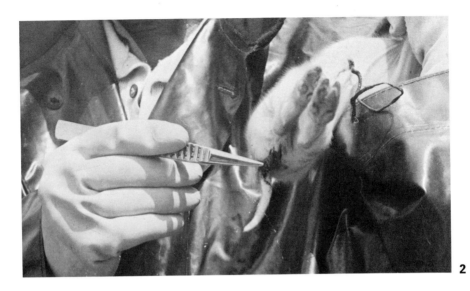

2

becomes dark and bloodstained *(photo 2)*: death soon follows.

What To Do About It

If ever you spot this bloodstained diarrhoea in the baby piglets get your veterinary surgeon on the job immediately. He will confirm the diagnosis by post-mortem examination *(photo 3)* and will prescribe immediate control.

Baby piglets will be given concentrated lamb dysentery anti-serum at birth and all the sows will be vaccinated with a specific vaccine. Within a short time the anti-serum can be discontinued because the vaccinated sows will pass on antibodies against the clostridium germ in their colostrum to the piglets.

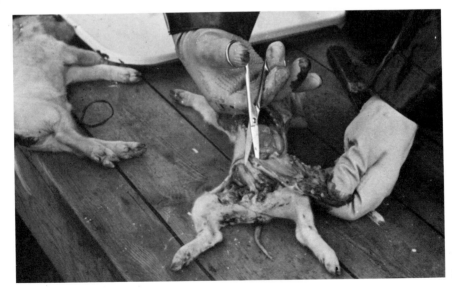

3

9
Joint-ill

JOINT-ILL *(photo 1)* in piglets is usually caused by one of the common germs, either a streptococcus or a staphylococcus—mostly by a streptococcus.

The 'bug' gains entrance through the piglet's navel *(photo 2)* during the first three days of life or through scratches or wounds caused by fighting. It usually takes two to three weeks to produce its effect. Round about that time it reaches the joints and starts to multiply, causing a painful inflammation and acute lameness. If untreated, pus forms in the joints within a day or two.

Obviously there must be a source of infection. Many adult sows are carriers of the streptococci and these bacteria can be inhaled by the piglets and gain

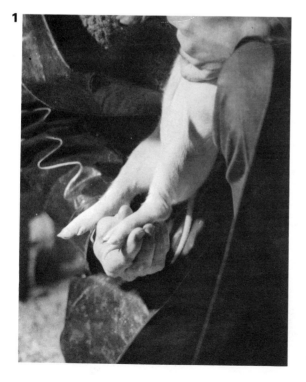

1

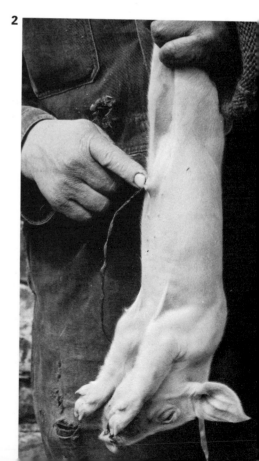

2

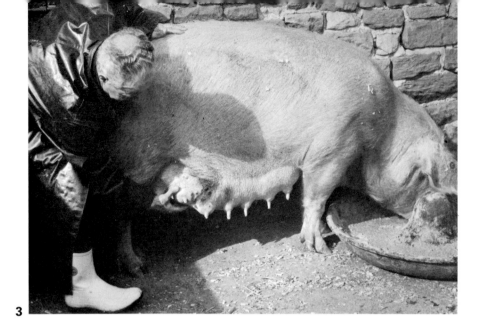

3

entry to the bloodstream via the tonsils. However, usually the source is a dirty floor in the farrowing pen; or perhaps a discharging abscess *(photo 3)* on the sow.

The first sign is lameness. The affected piglets (usually there are more than one) have difficulty in standing up and when they do they walk stiffly *(photo 4)*. They have a high temperature and stop suckling. Up to three quarters of the litter may be affected and if not treated early they die often showing brain symptoms—tremors, staggering and blindness.

Treatment

Fortunately, treatment, provided it is started early enough, is highly successful. The 'bugs' quickly succumb to antibiotics, but once the joints become markedly enlarged or the brain symptoms start treatment is of no avail.

4

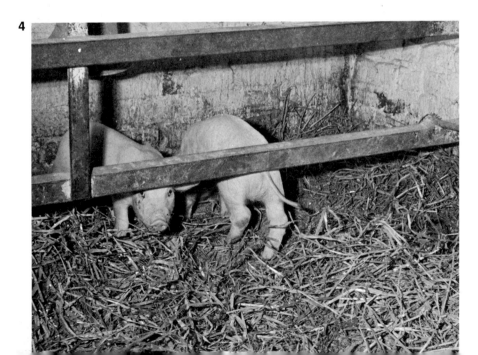

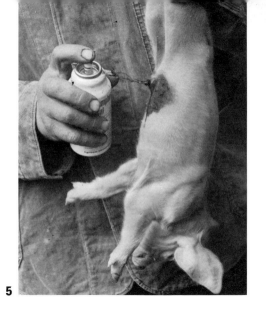

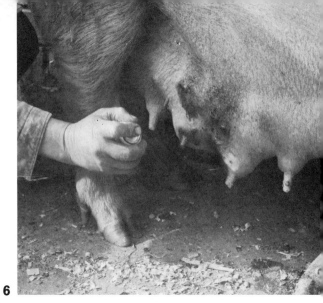

5

6

Prevention

Apart from the routine sterilisation of the farrowing pen in all herds where there is a history of joint-ill, it is wise to spray *(photo 5)* the navels of the piglets with a powerful antibiotic solution, once daily for the first three days of life.

At the same time check and make sure there are no discharging wounds or abscesses on the mother. If there are—bathe and dress them with the antibiotic spray *(photo 6)*.

Clip the baby piglet's incisor teeth *(photo 7)* at birth to avoid the facial and leg wounds caused by fighting.

Provide additional bedding at farrowing time to prevent knee damage to the piglets, another possible source of entry for the bacteria.

7

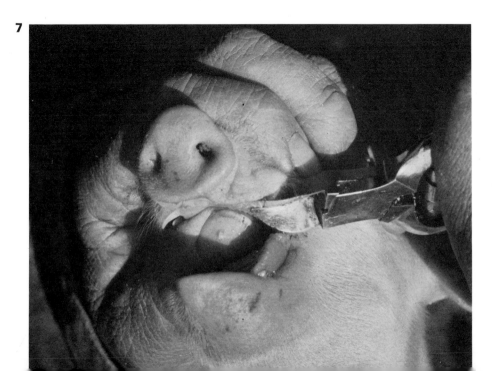

Streptococcal Meningitis in Older Pigs

This is an epidemic disease of weaned and fattening pigs which may flare up after mixing or moving.

Cause
The streptococcal bacilli are carried by recovered pigs (which are protected by natural immunity). These streptococci are spread to the unprotected pigs in the group via the respiratory system—that is, the victims actually breathe in the streptococci which invade the bloodstream via the tonsils.

Symptoms
The bacteria may take from 1 to 14 days to produce their effect.

The first sign of an outbreak may be the sudden death of a pig in good condition. Others in the batch will go off their feed and run a high temperature. If not treated immediately nervous symptoms soon appear, *viz.* staggering, paralysis, paddling, muscle spasms and death within 3 or 4 hours.

Treatment
Penicillin and other antibiotics given intramuscularly are specific but only if injected early before the nervous symptoms appear.

Prevention
Where the disease is established a broad spectrum antibiotic like amphicillin or tetracyclene in the drinking water is of considerable value but by no means infallible. All in-contact pigs may be protected by an intramuscular injection of long-acting penicillin. Commonsense cleanliness and husbandry at weaning time goes a long way towards effective control.

10
Non-infectious Diarrhoea

NON-INFECTIOUS diarrhoea is a mild scour *(photo 1)* seen usually in the biggest and healthiest piglets, and is due apparently to excess milk. The droppings are not unlike white cream.

What Should You Do About It?

Check the management. A few simple adjustments and a little bit of careful nursing are usually all that is necessary.

If the odd piglet dies then let your veterinary surgeon have it immediately to make sure that no bacteria are present.

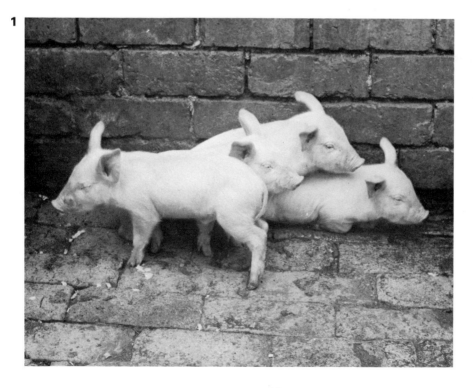

11
Two- to Three-week Scour

THIS type of scour *(photo 1)* occurs when the pigs are really getting on to creep feed and the antibodies acquired from the colostrum have not yet been reinforced by the antibodies from the young pigs' own bone marrow. If all the precautions I have just told you about have been rigidly adhered to, then the chances of getting this scour are not very great. But if the *E. coli* is very powerful or if the sows have not had sufficient time or opportunity to acquire the necessary resistance, then you may have to face it.

When it does occur the only way to deal

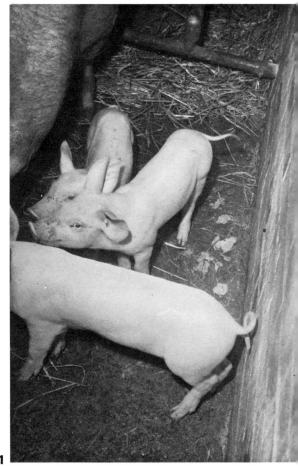

1

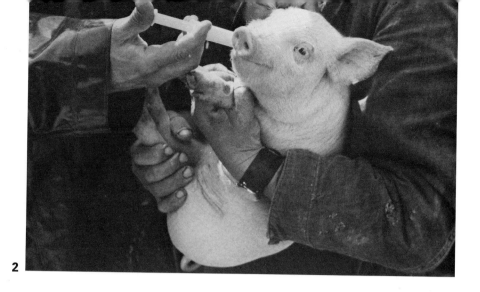

2

with it is to treat the individual pigs by giving specific antibiotics by mouth *(photo 2)*. Each piglet has to be caught and dosed with the requisite amount. Aim is merely to control the growth of the *E. coli* until the piglet's digestion has settled down and the antibody level has once more been built up.

Prevention

In addition to all the precautions outlined for baby piglet disease, scour at 2 to 3 weeks can be minimised if a really good creep food, containing a proportion of dried milk and low fibre, is provided. It is also less likely to occur if creep feeding is started early—say, at around 5 days, and *ad lib* fresh water *(photo 3)* is always available.

3

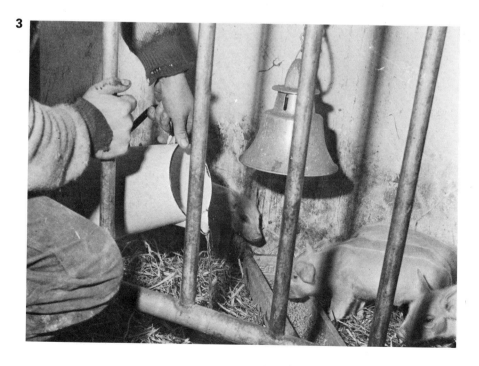

12
Transmissible Gastro-enteritis

TRANSMISSIBLE gastro-enteritis—or TGE—is a hyper-acute disease caused by a virus. It affects pigs of all ages and spreads alarmingly quickly throughout the entire herd. In general, the younger the pigs the more devastating is the disease: certainly it produces a high mortality in pigs under three weeks of age.

How To Spot The Disease
The first sign in the baby piglets is usually a profuse, foul-smelling, grey-greenish watery diarrhoea *(photo 1)*. The affected piglets vomit and show signs of extreme thirst. They literally 'dry up and die'.

In older pigs the signs are not so clear. There may be some diarrhoea, perhaps an occasional vomit but never any rise in temperature. The only sign

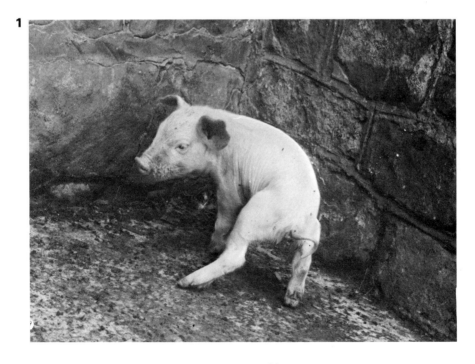

1

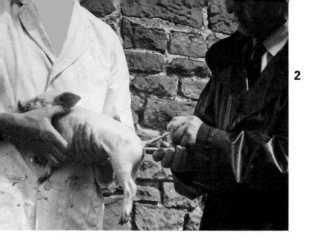

2

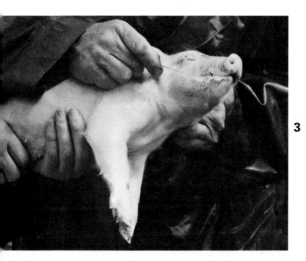

3

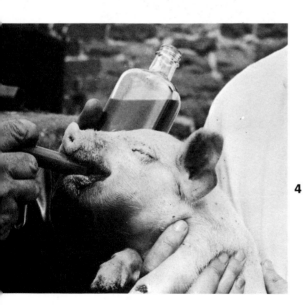

4

may be loss of appetite and of condition.

What To Do About It
TGE is definitely a problem for your veterinary surgeon *(photos 2 and 3)*. He will confirm the diagnosis on the symptoms and post-mortem findings.

Treatment
No drug is effective against the virus of TGE. The only effective treatment is the dosing *(photo 4)* of the affected piglets with citrated whole blood from recovered sows, but this is very much a matter for your veterinary surgeon.

Can TGE Be Prevented Or Controlled?
The disease fortunately, so far, is more or less confined to East Anglia and East Yorkshire, though it can break out suddenly in any herd. Birds are thought to be capable of spreading the virus.

Once the TGE has spread throughout a herd and done its damage it rarely flares up again—apparently because the recovered pigs develop a powerful immunity.

During an outbreak it is possible to exert some control by feeding the freshly-passed diarrhoeic faeces from the infected piglets mixed into the food of all the older pigs, but particularly the pregnant sows. Some immunity is established and transmitted to the new-born piglets in the sow's colostrum.

At the same time citrated whole blood from the recovered sows should be given daily by the mouth to all the susceptible piglets.

Research is proceeding and there is every prospect that an effective vaccine against transmissible gastro-enteritis will soon be available. So far however, no vaccine has been produced that will protect as well as natural infection. A dead vaccine available in the USA is relatively ineffective, though considerable success is now being claimed in the USA from the use of live vaccines.

13

Vomiting and Wasting Disease

THIS was thought to be a new disease introduced into our pig population from Canada, but examination of blood samples showed that it had been in the country for a number of years though we had not recognised it.

Cause
Definitely a virus.

Symptoms
It attacks piglets 10–14 days old. The first sign is vomiting. Affected piglets refuse to suckle, lie about, waste away and die. Oddly enough it rarely affects all the litter: on an average three piglets or up to three-quarters of the litter will die.

Unlike transmissible gastro-enteritis (TGE) it does not attack older pigs.

Treatment
There is no known treatment apart from good nursing—keeping the piglets warm and hoping for the best. Fortunately a fairly high degree of natural immunity follows an outbreak.

Prevention
There are some prospects that a vaccine may be developed against the virus, since immunity can be stimulated in non-pregnant gilts by feeding small portions of affected dead piglets.

As with all pig diseases it is advisable to keep a closed herd.

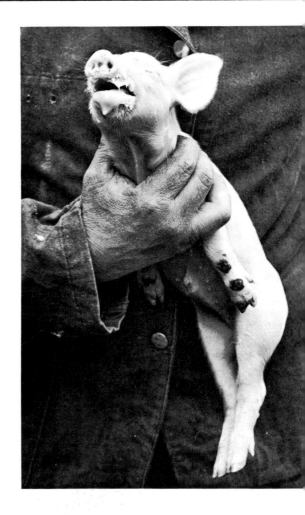

14
Infertility

HAVING survived the farrowing and reared the piglets, the next major headache is infertility. What constitutes infertility as a herd problem in a pig enterprise? Normally by natural service one could expect 80 per cent conception. If AI is being used then 60 to 70 per cent can be regarded as normal. If either of these figures drop by 10 per cent then you have an infertility problem.

What Causes Infertility?
I have found that the commonest causes are the simplest ones. For example:

1. The inability of the boar to insert his penis correctly. This is frequently due to foot trouble or other leg weaknesses, usually genetic in origin. It may also be due to too much work *(photo 1)* or to a young boar being bullied and knocked about when turned in with a bunch of adult sows; or the boar may be too small.

2. I have seen a fair bit of infertility secondary to and associated with *E. coli* metritis (up to 30 per cent).

3. Failure to serve at the correct time when using artificial insemination.

4. There is considerable evidence that gastro-intestinal worms in the sow will lead to infertility.

1
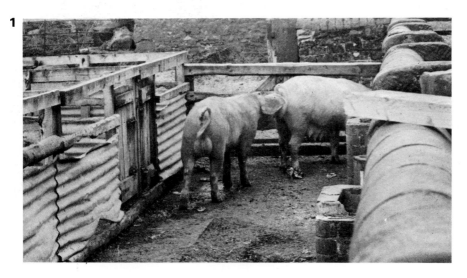

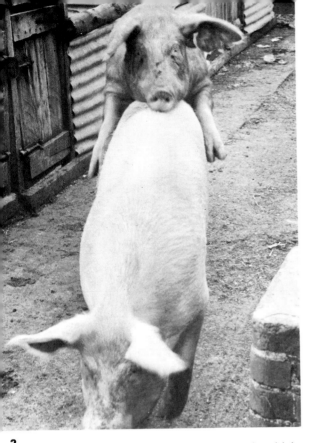

2

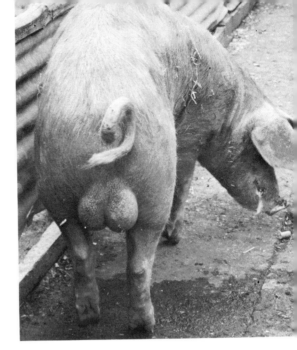

5. A disease called leptospirosis which may produce no other apparent symptoms but can cause wholesale infertility in the herd.

6. Age can be a factor in fertility, particularly in gilts. Puberty is reached usually when they are about 200 lb in weight and they reach their maximum fertility on the third observable heat period, generally when they are around 260–280 lb in weight.

7. Diseases like parvovirus etc.

How To Tackle The Problem

I suggest you consult your veterinary surgeon who in turn may well bring in a specialist.

There are, however, a few sensible general precautions:

1. Restrict the boar to between 3 and 4 services weekly *(photo 2)*.

2. Keep his feet in good order by regular exercise on concrete *(photo 3)* and pay prompt attention to any lameness. Also make sure the boar is big enough for the job.

3. Observe high standards of feeding and cleanliness with both sows and boars.

4. Dose the sows with one of the many excellent modern worm remedies *(photo 4)*. I am convinced that we still have a great deal to learn about gastro-intestinal parasites in pigs and I feel certain that it is essential to dose, as a routine, all sows as well as the piglets at weaning time. This is often forgotten with disastrous effects on both the condition and longevity of the sow herd. Powerful anthelmintic injections are now available, as are in-feed anthelmintics.

5. Vaccinate sows, gilts and boars against parvovirus (see page 20).

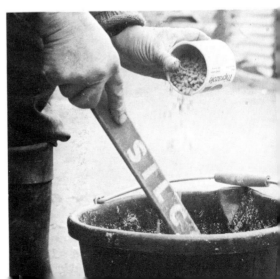

15
Anoestrus

ANOESTRUS means when the gilts or sows do not come in season *(photo 1)*.

Causes
- Protein deficiency.
- Deficiency of vitamin A.
- Intensive management.
- Hormonal upset.

Treatment
Obviously a job for the veterinary surgeon since the cause has to be diagnosed before the cure can be prescribed.

I have always had best results by giving injections of 1,500 international units of pregnant mare's serum *(photo 2)* followed a week later by 1,000 international units of luteinising hormone. A very useful practical hint to cure anoestrus in gilts is to put two newly-weaned sows with them; within a few days of the sows coming in season the gilts will start plainly showing.

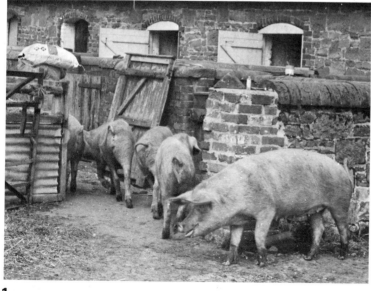

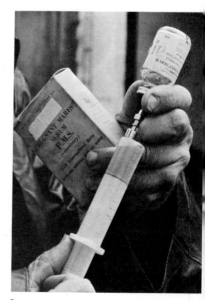

1

2

DISEASES OF WEANERS AND OLDER PIGS

1
Preventing Stress

STRESS factors, especially at weaning time, include:
- Actual movement of the pigs from one pen to another *(photo 1)*.
- Handling involved in such movement.
- Psychological effect of strange surroundings.
- Changed environment involving different atmospheric conditions and contact with a new set of bacteria. This is especially the case when the

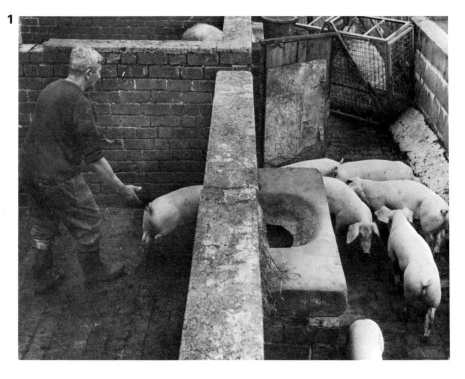

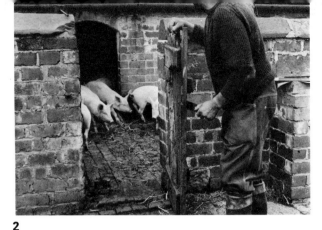

2

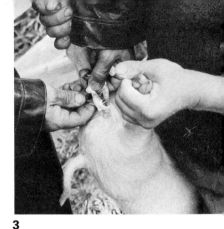

3

follow-on pens are dirty and draughty *(photo 2)*.

- Castration *(photo 3)*.
- Worming.
- Washing for mange *(photo 4)*.
- Vaccination.
- Weighing.
- Changes in the diet *(photo 5)*.
- Running weaned litters with other litters weaned at the same time. When this is done the freshly-weaned pigs have to combat attacks from strange bacteria at a time when they are least able to stand up to them.

Remember that any stress factor at weaning time can lead to diarrhoea, bowel oedema or death. If you are not prepared to take implicit care to avoid all these factors then you mustn't expect drugs to do the job for you. Drugs, especially antibiotics, are never any more than a very poor substitute for good husbandry: they should never be resorted to or even considered unless or until all the husbandry faults have been rectified.

The routine I advise at weaning time is as follows:

1. Wean late. I'd say an absolute minimum of 5 weeks and as near 8 weeks as possible *(photo 6)*. In fact in some particularly badly-affected herds the problems have disappeared when the weaning period has been increased to 9 weeks. Certainly the earlier the weaning the greater chance of trouble.

2. If possible leave the weaners in the same pen for the whole of their fattening life. It this is not practical then keep them in the pen for at least 2 weeks.

3. Always remove the sow from the piglets at weaning and never vice versa. Take the sow away completely *(photo 7)*. Gradual weaning is time-consuming and has no apparent advantage.

4. Castrate at 3 weeks (or better still—don't castrate).

5. Vaccinate at least one full week before weaning.

6. Worm and wash for mange 2 weeks after weaning *(photo 8)*.

7. In fact the only handling stress I per-

4

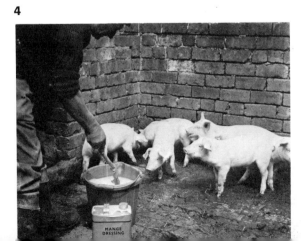

5

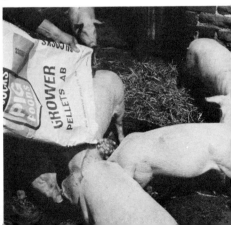

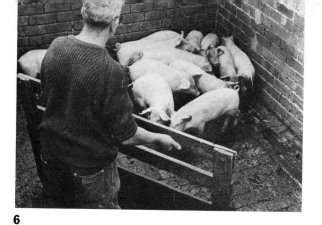

6

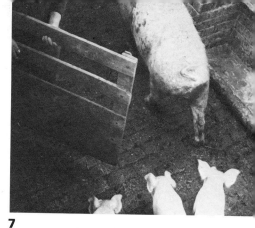

7

mit at weaning time is weighing *(photo 9)*
and even then I prefer to see that done
later.

8. Make sure that the pigs are eating,
before weaning, exactly the same food as
they are going to get subsequently *(photo
10)*. In this way the only dietetical change
will be loss of the sow's milk. Keeping the
weaners on identical food is simple and
yet, again and again, I see this precaution
neglected.

9. Avoid grouping of litters or, if this
isn't practical, postpone grouping until
the pigs are at least 10 weeks old.

10. Careful observation of these simple
husbandry factors at weaning comprises
preventative medicine of the highest order.

11. Where the management and feeding
are first class, then 3 week weaning is successful provided all other precautions are
observed.

8

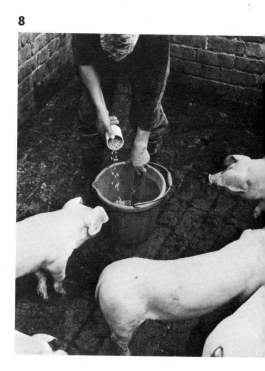

9

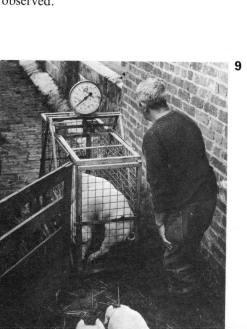

10

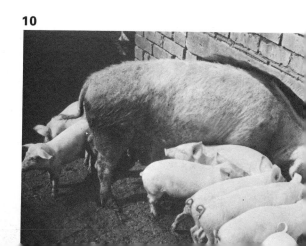

2
Bowel Oedema

ONE of our most constant killers is bowel oedema where the best pigs, usually freshly weaned, are found dead or staggering about like drunken men with their eyelids swollen up *(photo 1)* just as though they'd had a night on the tiles!

Cause

Once again thought to be the *E. coli* 'bug', though scientists are still arguing about exactly how the effects are produced. Predisposing cause seems to be stress, produced by castration, inoculation, transport, change in environment, and most common of all, changes in feeding— especially if sow nuts are suddenly fed *(photo 2)* because the growers pellets or meal is temporarily out of stock. Anapylaxis (shock), allergy and virus infection have all been blamed.

Treatment

Whenever there is an outbreak of oedema treat all the weaners on the farm identically by withholding food for 12 hours, at the same time providing ample warm water to drink *(photo 3)*. Afterwards, feed in gradually increasing quantities an easily digestible feed such as a warm mash of bran and sharps. After 2 or 3 days of mashes the diet can gradually be returned to normal.

Sulphonamides, furazolidone and antibiotics can be fed but I've found them expensive and of little real value.

1

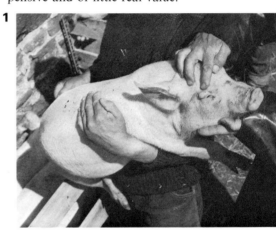

2

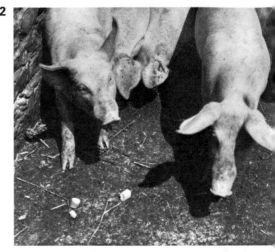

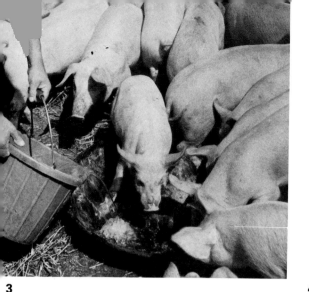

3

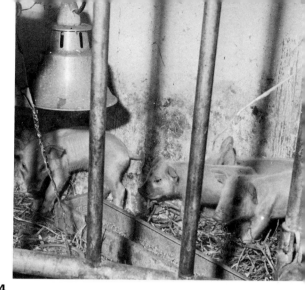

4

Prevention

Obviously, prevention is a much better idea—here is the routine I recommend:

1. Start creep-feeding the piglets at 5 days old and at the same time provide fresh, clean, warm water daily *(photo 4)*.

2. At weaning keep the piglets on exactly the same creep feed for at least 10 days and make sure the water supply is still ample, clean and warm.

3. If possible leave the piglets in the same environment during this period of change. In other words, take the sow away *(photo 5)* from the piglets instead of the traditional vice versa.

4. Don't—whatever you do—overfeed. It's much better to keep the little beggars short for a day or two *(photo 6)*.

5. Keep the troughs and feed buckets spotlessly cleaned *(photo 7)*.

If you do all this and still get oedema then it's a job for your veterinary surgeon.

5

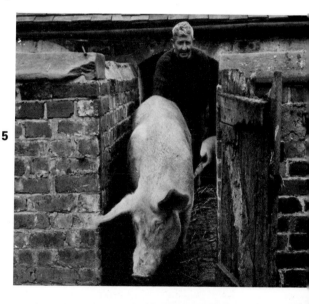

6

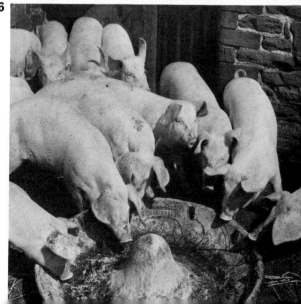

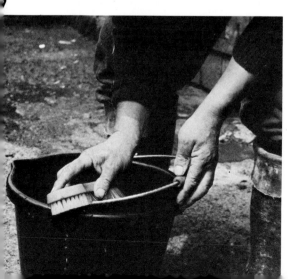

3
Salt Poisoning

SALT poisoning *(photo 1)* is an almost identical condition to oedema which, in fact, it is often diagnosed as. It is, however, not usually due to feeding excess salt but simply to not providing sufficient water to dilute the salt content of the food.

Symptoms
Affected pigs suddenly stand still with a strained tense expression, and within a few minutes start champing their jaws and frothing at the mouth. Their bodies

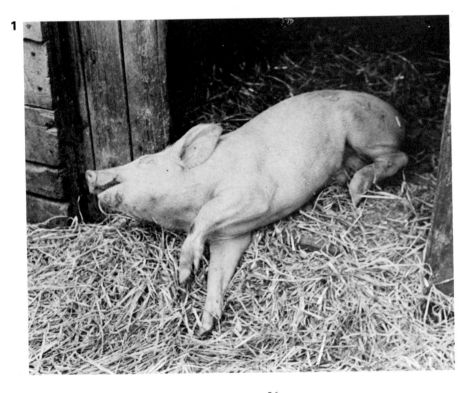

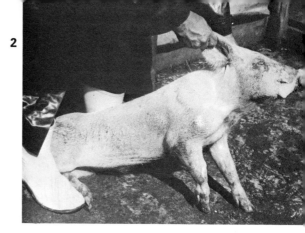

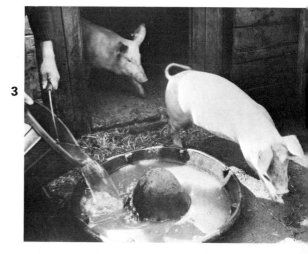

quiver and they run backwards to collapse in a epileptic fit *(photo 2)*. The fits recur every few minutes, and in the intervals between the pigs blunder blindly about or stand pressing the head or nose against the wall.

Treatment

If ever these symptoms appear an immediate increase in the water supply *(photo 3)* will produce spectacular results—I've seen a pen of drunken, semi-blind pigs drain a trough of water and walk steadily almost within minutes.

Prevention

Prevention is simple: if you have to move your weaners from the sow to a strange pen, don't rely on water bowls—provide open water troughs for at least the first week *(photo 4)*. It takes at least three or four days for the shy pigs to get used to drinking from a strange bowl and during that period water deficiency spells—death.

The more modern water dispensers can take longer to get used to (see coloured illustration facing page 65).

When salty rations such as whey and buttermilk are fed, the drinking water *must* be provided *ad lib*. (i.e. in open troughs).

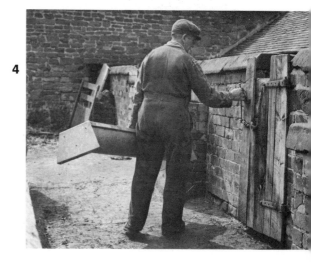

4
Post-weaning Scours

POST-WEANING scour is second in economic importance to the 2- to 3-day-old scours I told you about earlier. It can and does cause tremendous losses not only in actual deaths but in wasted food through subsequent unthriftiness. This happens in the best of herds and often hits the best pigs *(photo 1)* within 10 days of weaning. The diarrhoeic faeces are grey or brown, watery but no trace of blood. The temperature may rise for several days.

Cause
Once again *E. coli* is involved. And once again prevention, as with the baby piglets, must be aimed at building up the natural resistance, and lowering the available doses of the bacteria.

But even more important in preventing this post-weaning scour is absolute care with the feeding and management at weaning time.

1
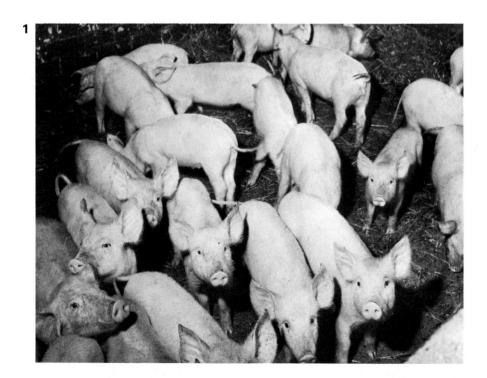

Drill To Follow

1. When weaning, take the sow *(photo 2)* from the piglets (as recommended in the prevention of oedema) and leave the piglets on ad lib creep feed and ample warm water *for at least a week*, preferably 10 days to a fortnight.

2. After a week introduce—mixed with the creep—the growers' meal gradually, and progressively aim at a full replacement of the creep after 12 to 14 days. If at this stage you change the diet suddenly then you're asking for trouble and you'll most certainly get it.

3. If the scours do appear a light laxative diet *(photo 3)* containing 3 to 4 per cent of dried yeast is more vital than the use of drugs. Remember drugs can never repair bowel damage.

4. If post-weaning scour is a major problem in your herd and you are not prepared to take the strict husbandry precautions I recommend, then drugs are probably of more use if given as a prophylactic in the drinking water—say at 4–5 days before weaning up to two weeks after weaning. But remember! This is only another substitute for good husbandry and in the long run drugs will only lead you into more serious trouble by creating resistant strains of coli.

5. Probably better than drugs is the comparatively new oral vaccine, but your veterinary surgeon will advise on this. (Intagen in creep and/or weaner rations.)

6. Routine vaccination of the breeding sows: again under veterinary supervision.

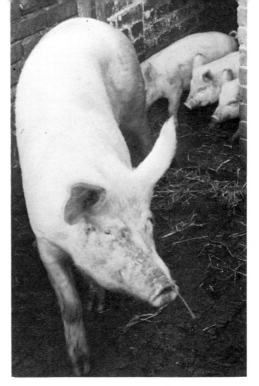

2

3

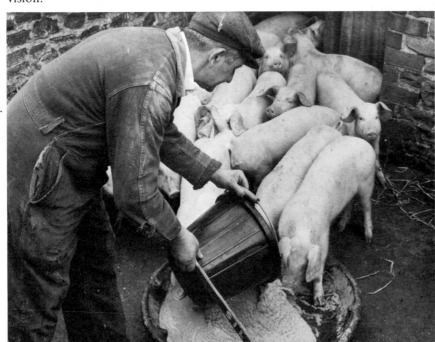

5
Swine Dysentery

THIS DISEASE which attacks mainly pigs between the ages of 7–16 weeks occurs all over the world and is very common in Britain. It can be very severe in *sows* at or near farrowing and can lead to sudden death.

Cause

Originally swine dysentery was thought to be caused by a vibrio coli organism or a leptospira but it is now established that the primary cause is a large spirochaete with the highly scientific name of *treponema hyodysenteriae*. For the purpose of this book the name is of academic significance only.

How It Spreads

Swine dysentery is spread to healthy pigs when they eat food or bedding contaminated by the faeces of affected or 'carrier' animals. The 'carriers' are able to spread the disease for at least 90 days after they have apparently recovered. The spirochaete may take from 7 to 60 days to produce its effect in a victim.

Predisposing Causes

Similar stress factors to those described in post-weaning scour. In my experience the two most common are first of all a lack of hygiene and secondly the routine feeding of antibiotics. Normally the spirochaete grows only with difficulty

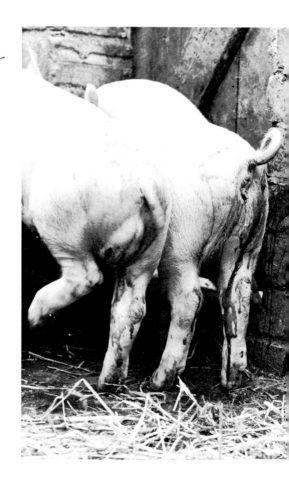

because of the general bacterial screen in the pigs intestine. The antibiotics,

60

especially if fed over a fairly long period, say 14 days or more, destroy most of the bowel's bacterial resistance and encourage the spirochaete and other bacteria such as the vibrio and leptospira to grow.

Symptoms

Affected pigs go off their feed. The temperature rises to 104°–105°F for about 24 hours then it returns to normal (102·5°F) as soon as the diarrhoea starts. Of course in a large unit the diarrhoea may be the first symptoms noted.

Blood and mucus appear in the diarrhoeic dung which is at first yellowish in colour but later brownish-red, liquid and foul smelling.

If untreated, the patients rapidly become thin with sunken eyes, rough coat, hollow flanks and prominent ribs and spine. If treated late some may remain stunted with chronic diarrhoea.

Treatment

In all outbreaks it is best to consult your veterinary surgeon who has a wide variety of effective drugs at his disposal. He will prescribe and change the drugs according to circumstances since the spirochaete builds up a resistance to any one drug used over a prolonged period.

Prevention and Control

As with post-weaning scour and all other bacterial infections, essential preventative measures are good housing and first class management. If at all possible avoid feeding antibiotics at weaning time.

Treat suspect outbreaks promptly in consultation with the veterinary surgeon and take his advice on general control measures. He will probably advise precautionary medication of the feed or drinking water for all bought in pigs until the disease is under control.

After treating infected pigs I usually recommend a thorough cleansing and disinfection of their pen plus a 14-day pig-free rest for the pen before restocking if this is at all practical.

Leptospirosis

Infection with spirochaetes of the Leptospira species may produce no apparent symptoms or it may cause fever, jaundice and death in piglets and abortion and stillbirths in sows. It occurs worldwide and particularly in pigs kept outside.

How Do Pigs Become Infected?

By ingestion of food or water contaminated by rats. The spirochaete can also gain entry through wounds and is passed on to the piglets through the placenta (i.e. in the uterus or womb).

Symptoms

As above with the majority of pigs showing no clinical signs. The acute cases usually occur in piglets and these show a rise in temperature to up to nearly 106°F, diarrhoea, jaundice and in most cases death.

In sows the abortions are usually accompanied by a high temperature, loss of milk and jaundice.

Treatment

Broad spectrum antibiotics as prescribed by a veterinary surgeon.

Prevention

In breeding herds where leptospirosis has been diagnosed the sows can be protected by vaccinating before service.

As always hygiene and strict cleanliness play an important part in control.

Recent research has shown that a commercial product called *Antec Farm Fluid S* diluted to one in 400 of hard water completely destroys the primary causal agent of swine dysentery in highly infective faeces.

6

Salmonellosis

Salmonellosis is a comparatively uncommon disease of pigs with only approximately 200 outbreaks a year among British swine.

Cause
Several strains of Salmonella organisms. At one time a particular strain the *Salmonella cholerae suis* caused at least half of the pig outbreaks, but lately the majority of British outbreaks are due to the *Salmonella typhimurium* which is carried by rats. At least 2 other salmonellae have been implicated.

When Do The Salmonellae Attack?
Pigs of all ages can be affected although outbreaks occur most frequently in pigs aged between 3 and 4 months *(photo 1)* at which age septicaemia is more likely.

How To Recognise Salmonellosis
Since salmonellosis is often an acute blood poisoning the affected pigs run high temperatures and there is marked reddening or purpling of the skin of the ears *(photo 2)*, belly and top of the legs. Such cases die within 24 hours.

Where the bowel only is infected (the acute enteric form) there is a thin watery diarrhoea and the temperature rises to between 105°F and 107°F. This leads to general weakness, tremors, paralysis and occasionally pneumonia.

Occasionally a more chronic disease occurs characterised by intermittent fever, diarrhoea and progressive emaciation. The persistent diarrhoea

1
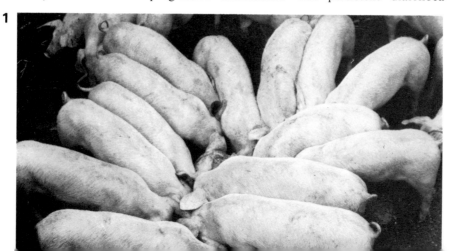

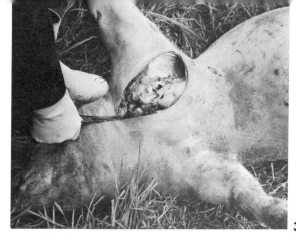

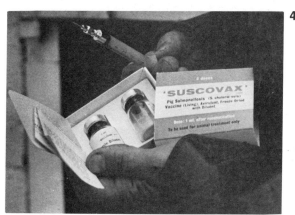

3

4

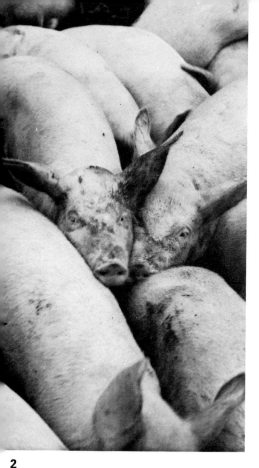

2

may contain shreds of bowel lining but rarely blood. If such cases do survive they remain unthrifty.

What To Do About It

Consult your veterinary surgeon immediately. He will confirm the diagnosis by faecal swabs or on post-mortem examination *(photo 3)*. It is of tremendous importance that this disease should be diagnosed correctly because recovered pigs can remain 'carriers', passing the salmonella germs out in their dung and continually infecting new pens and fresh ground. Even adult sows and gilts may pick up the 'bug' and transmit it to younger more susceptible pigs without showing any signs of the disease whatsoever.

Can It Be Treated?

In my experience no treatment is effective against the acute septicaemic salmonellosis.

In the more chronic type, sulpha drugs, nitrofurans and certain antibiotics do have some beneficial effect. However, it is very doubtful if treatment of salmonellosis in the pig is ever economical. I would not recommend it. It is much better to make sure of the diagnosis, then to concentrate on preventative measures.

Prevention

1. Wherever possible buy weaners and stores from known clean sources, vaccinate on arrival at the farm and isolate for one month.

2. Liaise with your veterinary surgeon and if the infection is due to Cholerae suis, vaccinate *(photo 4)* all piglets between the ages of 2–6 weeks, certainly at least a week before moving the weaners to a fattening house.

3. Observe carefully the usual commonsense hygiene precautions.

63

7
Clostridium Infection

THIS DISEASE is caused by two germs *viz.* the *Clostridium chauvoei* and the clostridium oedematiens (*C. Novyi*) and can only be diagnosed by a veterinary surgeon on post-mortem.

What Type of Pig Does It Affect?
Fattening pigs getting towards pork or bacon *(photo 1)*.

How Does It Affect Them?
Sudden death *(photo 2)* followed by extremely rapid putrefaction.

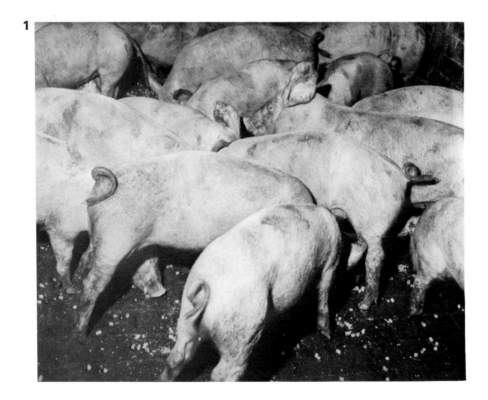

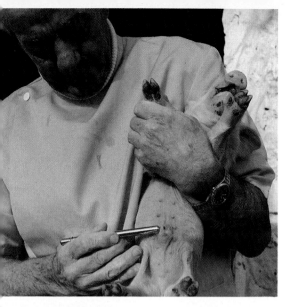

The joint ill and tetanus bacteria gain entrance through the piglet's navel during the first 3 days of life or through scratches or wounds caused by fighting. Symptoms of joint ill do not appear until 2 or 3 weeks later (pages 37 and 67).

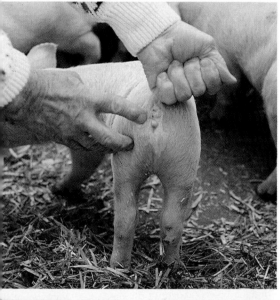

Three-week-old scour, which occurs when the pigs are getting on to creep feed and the antibodies acquired from the colostrum have not yet been reinforced by the antibodies from the young pig's own bone marrow (page 42).

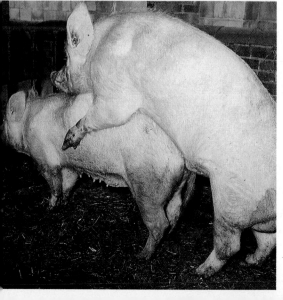

To avoid the problem of infertility, restrict the boar to 3 or 4 services weekly (page 47).

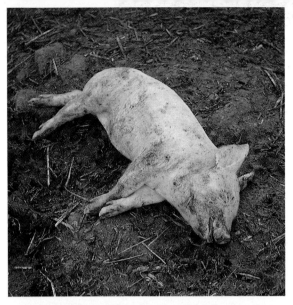

A pig dying from salt poisoning which is usually due to not providing sufficient water to dilute the salt content in the food.

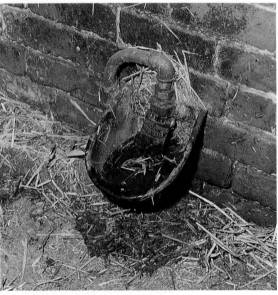

Ample water supply is vital, be it from the old-fashioned drinking bowls (above) or the more up to date dispensers (below) (page 57).

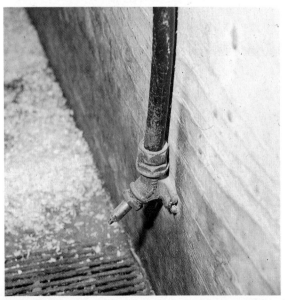

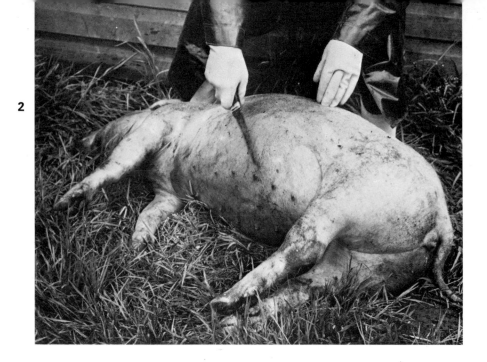

Where Does It Come From?
The bowel of the pig.

What Causes It To Flare Up?
Alterations in the consistency of the food *(photo 3)*. This can occur when the screen in the hammer-mill becomes worn *(photo 4)*; larger particles of meal are churned out and these upset the digestive process.

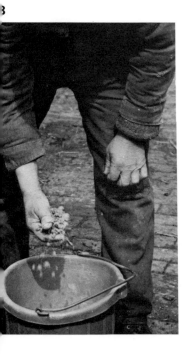

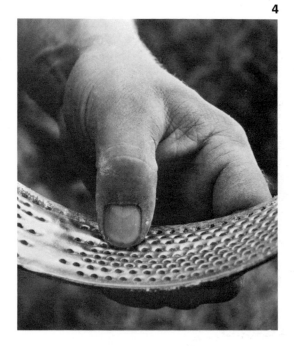

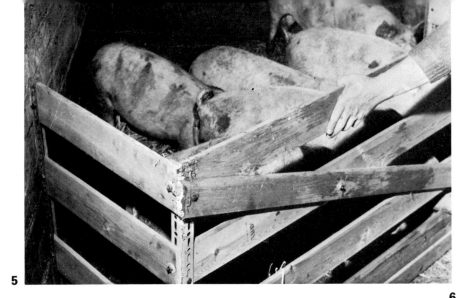

5

6

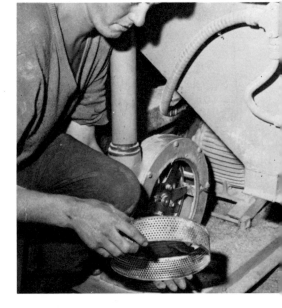

Another stress factor involved in this condition is when the pigs are handled *(photo 5)* or confined in a hot *dry* atmosphere. Pigs have no sweat glands and no adequate heat-regulating mechanism. They can't get rid of the heat so they literally boil up inside and this produces conditions ideal for the growth of the *Clostridia*.

How To Prevent Losses
- Check the mechanism of your mill and mixer at least once a month *(photo 6)*.
- Take great care to avoid overcrowding *(photo 7)* or handling in a hot dry atmosphere. You may get away with it in a hot moist atmosphere such as prevails in a sweat-box piggery, but never subject a fattening pig to the stress of a hot *dry* environment.
- Vaccines are available.

7

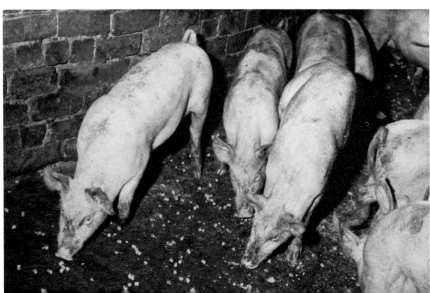

Tetanus

One other Clostridial bacterium can attack pigs at any age, *viz*. the *Clostridium tetani* which causes tetanus.

The bacteria gain entry through the navel or via castration or other wounds.

Symptoms
Stiffness, abnormal gait, muscle spasms and death. Clinical signs appear a few days to weeks after wound infection. Within 24–28 hours the muscles stiffen, the ears are held erect, the tail straight and finally rigid paralysis sets in. Any noise produces tetanic spasms.

Treatment
Muscle relaxants and penicillin. Prognosis not good.

Prevention
Care and hygiene at castration time. Vaccination is possible but impractical. With modern methods of feeding castration is no longer necessary and has been largely abandoned in many enterprises.

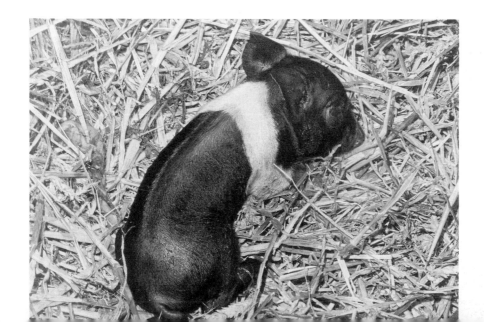

8

Enzootic Pneumonia *(Virus Pneumonia)*

FRANKLY, I think it's fair to say that nowadays there is no excuse for any self-contained pig unit to be plagued with virus pneumonia. After all, the routine for the clearance of a herd is quite straightforward and easy to apply.

Yet VPP remains a hazard, especially in commercial fattening units where weaners are bought from many and varied sources. A hazard which not only costs life but which hinders growth rate and wastes countless tons of expensive feeding-stuffs.

For pig farmers who are not virus-free there are two alternative methods of fighting virus pneumonia:

1. Empty all the houses.
Clean, disinfect *(photo 1)* and leave empty for at least three weeks then stock up from virus-free sources.

2. A second-best, but perhaps more practical, solution is to improve the housing so that virus pneumonia then ceases to be an economic problem.

We must never forget that the course VPP takes depends entirely on environment.

The ideal environment for fattening pigs is one which provides a constant warm temperature in the sleeping quarters and a simultaneous supply of fresh air. To obtain this the owner must make the sleeping pens compact, draught-proof, insulated and, to some extent, isolated.

It's easy to do this in any house if one simple fact is borne in mind—the only way to make any pen draught-proof is to close it completely over the top and on three sides *(photo 2)*. That is all any practical man needs to know—his common sense and ingenuity will do the rest.

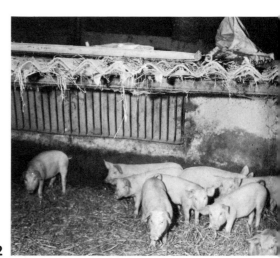

1   2

In most houses it simply means constructing draught-proof kennels *(photo 3)* or each pen within the main building. If you want to find out if your efforts are successful try sleeping with the pigs! In an ideal kennel you should be able to lie comfortably without blankets.

Virus pneumonia is caused by a very minute germ which scientists now believe must be a mycoplasma, though they are not quite sure about it. Large numbers of these minute germs invade the small cells which lie just underneath the lining of the pig's bronchi, causing the cells to swell and push the bronchial lining inwardly. This, in turn, causes a constriction of the bronchial tubes, and makes the pig cough mechanically.

It's easy to understand, therefore, why a virus pneumonia cough is harsh and dry, with little or no sputum—since there is no sputum or pus at the source of infection. It is also interesting and important to note that, in the early stages at any rate, so-called virus pneumonia is not a pneumonia at all, but merely a mechanical bronchitis. The germs spread to the lungs only very slowly, and only when the pig's resistance is lowered by the effects of bad housing.

Even then, although there is an area of damaged lung tissue, it is not by any means an acute pneumonia, and will not, in itself, kill the pig.

It is an acute secondary bacterial pneumonia which causes death. But, again, this only sets in when the environmental conditions are bad—when the house is draughty, cold, damp or subjected to any extremes of temperatures. The bacteria then launch themselves from the virus site, and invade the neighbouring lung tissue.

When the germ is introduced into a virus-free herd, it is thought to flare up into a fatal pneumonia more readily, especially in baby pigs 10–20 days old. But this does not happen if the pig's environment is good—only if the housing is bad will the bacteria really go to town.

Clients often ask me where the germ of virus pneumonia come from. The answer is that the 'bugs' come from infected pigs which we call 'carriers' *(photo 4)*.

Here it is important to remember that young pigs are the most likely carriers because, after 12 months, an immunity is developed and the carrier danger decreases with age. The disease is spread by direct contact of carriers with healthy pigs, and only very rarely via the boots or clothing. This is an interesting fact not generally appreciated.

Outside the pig the virus lives only for a very short time, so that any pen will be clear after being empty for a few days. Sunshine, drying, and disinfectant rapidly kill the 'bug'.

Antibiotic injections are only of use in combating the secondary bacterial pneumonia.

One of the most severe secondary bacterial pneumonias is that caused by a bacterium called the *Pasteurella multocida* producing a pneumonia which we call Pasteurellosis.

This may also flare up after any of the other swine respiratory problems.

3

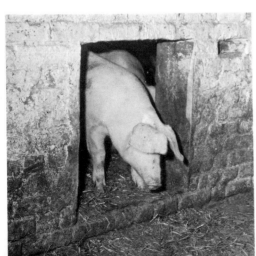

4

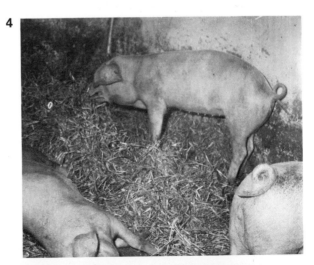

No known drug will have any direct effect on the virus once it's inside the pig. The logical way to fight the virus, therefore, is to eliminate it, if at all possible.

Here is what I have found to be a practical plan for eliminating the 'bug' and building up a virus-free herd.

The ideal animals to start with are the older sows *(photo 5)*. This means those that have had at least three litters, because, as I mentioned earlier, the older they get the more immune they become and the less likely they are to be carriers.

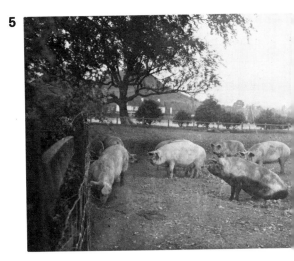

Of course this is grand, especially for the pedigree breeders, because the old sows are invariably the best, and are of known breeding potential. The pick of the old sows should be farrowed and kept in isolation, either in insulated arks in the field, away from all contact with infected pigs, or in a separate building.

Weaned pigs from them should be housed for 4 weeks, and then, if free from coughing, one or two of the hogs should be sacrificed as porkers, and their lungs sent to a laboratory for microscopical examination. This is the only way mild cases can be spotted.

It is essential to be absolutely ruthless— if the lungs show the slightest sign of infection, the whole litter should be scrapped. If clear, they should be kept, and thus gradually a virus-free herd will be built up. With care and luck, the job can be done in 2 years.

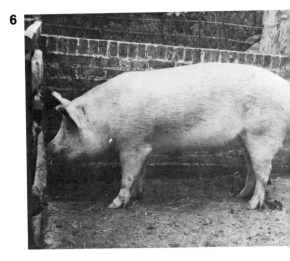

An old boar *(photo 6)* may be used with reasonable safety—the older the better. But, if available, artificial insemination is probably preferable.

9
Other Respiratory Diseases

APART from enzootic pneumonia (formerly known as virus pneumonia) it is vital to record the other known infections of the pig's respiratory passages if only because respiratory disease causes $7\frac{1}{2}$ per cent of the total deaths in pigs up to 3 weeks of age and $12\frac{1}{2}$ per cent of deaths from 3 to 8 weeks.

There are six other respiratory diseases of pigs. Three affect the upper air passages and three the lungs. In the upper passages there occur:

Inclusion Body Rhinitis. This affects baby piglets *(photo 1)* particularly. It produces sneezing and snuffling and a death rate of up to 100 per cent. It is caused by a virus.

Atrophic Rhinitis. This affects pigs of all ages and leads to watery eyes, distorted noses and wheezing *(photo 2)*. Atrophic rhinitis is now known to be triggered off by a calcium deficiency. This leads to a disintegration of the turbinate bones inside the pig's nasal cavities and a secondary bacterial infection flares up in the damaged turbinates.

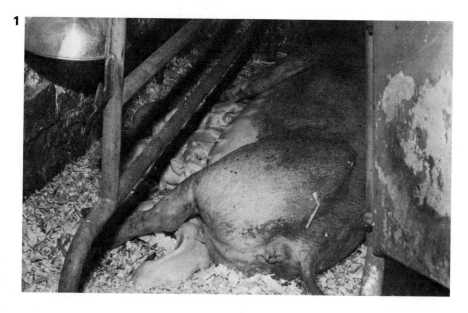
1

Infectious Rhinitis. This is an inflammation of the lining membranes of the upper respiratory tract. It is caused by bacteria and produces coughing and sneezing. It is extremely common and rarely fatal, though it does produce unthrifty litters.

In the lungs there occur:

Swine Influenza. A bacterial bronchopneumonia reported mainly in Europe. It has not been officially recognised in Britain during the last 20 years but I personally feel it occurs and is passed off by practitioners as enzootic pneumonia.

Ascaris. The larvae or intermediate stages of the Ascaris (roundworm) migrate through the lungs and produce small haemorrhages. Bacteria move in and a secondary pneumonia is the result.

Moreover, metastrongyle worms which live and breed in the lungs of the pig can and do produce a nasty pneumonia. These adult lung worms may appear in the lungs from 10 weeks onwards. They cause persistent coughing and unthriftiness.

Giant-cell pneumonia, a comparatively newly-recognised condition, which is hereditary, and usually fatal. In addition to the pneumonia the affected piglets show abnormal or clubbed feet and usually break out in a skin rash (*Vegetative Dermatosis*). The rash suddenly appears when the piglets are 2 or 3 days old. The piglets don't thrive and a fatal pneumonia usually sets in when they are 6 or 7 weeks old.

Prevention And Control

As in enzootic pneumonia, environment is all-important. Constant temperatures, freedom from draught, insulated floors *(photo 3)*—in fact, a liberal use of common sense will do more to control respiratory infections than any drugs.

Lung worms rarely present a problem where regular and efficient dosing against bowel worms (ascaris) is practised.

To sum up, therefore, good housing and sound husbandry are our main defences against respiratory diseases of pigs.

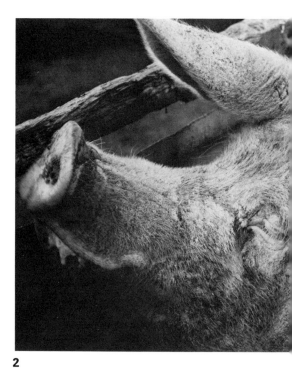

2

3

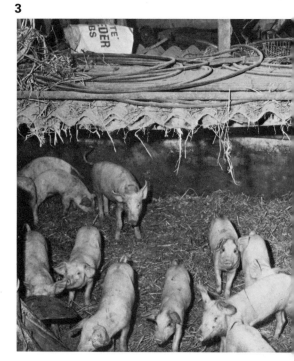

Infectious Atrophic Rhinitis

This is the only type that can or should be treated and whether to embark on a comprehensive treatment programme depends on the severity of the condition. I have found it advantageous to treat subacute and acute outbreaks.

In the subacute there are intermittent sneezing attacks in most litters with persistent though occasional coughing eventually leading to pneumonia. Inevitably the conversion rate is adversely affected.

In the acute outbreaks the persistent sneezing leads to nasal discharge and nose bleeds in both weaners and porkers, twisted snouts, more frequent pneumonias, general unthriftiness and in unprotected gilts and sows abortions and stillbirths.

The secondary bacteria involved are called *Bordetella bronchiseptica*.

Treatment
a. Long acting, broad spectrum antibiotic injections to the suckling piglets.

b. Antibiotics and/or sulphonamides in the food (both the creep and the adult feed). At the same time consult the feed merchant's nutrition adviser to make sure there is the correct ratio of calcium and phosphorus and adequate vitamin D_3 in the ration.

In subacute attacks
A check on the nutrition and the feed medication are probably sufficient.

Prevention And Control
a. Of prime importance—first-class housing and management (as with all respiratory diseases).

b. Routine medication of the creep and adult feed with sulphonamides, etc. (Suitable drugs will be prescribed by the veterinary surgeon.)

c. Routine injections of piglets with long-acting antibiotic at 3 days, 10 days and 3 weeks.

d. The use of one of several available vaccines (again the veterinary surgeon will advise).

10
Erysipelas

SWINE ERYSIPELAS is caused by a bacterium called *Erysipelothrix insidiosa*, several strains of which occur.

Where Does It Come From?
The erysipelas germ lives in the tonsils and various glands throughout the pig's body and is passed out intermittently in the urine and dung *(photo 1)*. A large percentage of completely normal pigs are 'carriers' of the 'bug'. Also the organism can survive on the ground for long periods.

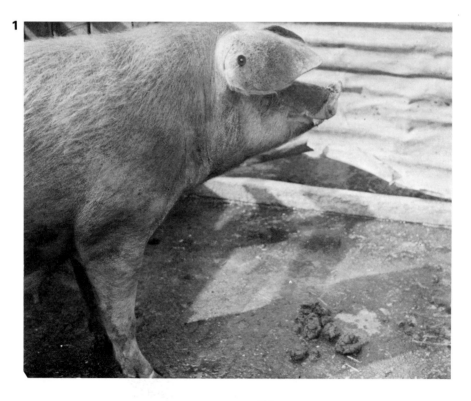

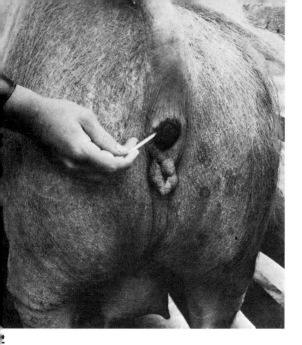

What Causes It To Flare Up?

Hot humid weather seems to favour the growth of the germ and acute erysipelas is most common in summer. Stress due to viral infection, fatigue, pregnancy, vaccination etc. can also predispose.

Symptoms

There are three types of erysipelas:

- Acute.
- Subacute.
- Chronic.

Acute. This form is easily recognised. The pig, usually one of the older ones, goes off its food, runs a very high temperature or around 107° or 108° F, and breaks out in raised reddish or purplish blotches. The high fever causes severe constipation *(photo 2)*.

Subacute. In my experience swine erysipelas manifests itself chiefly in the subacute form. The outstanding symptom (and very often the only one) is lameness or stiffness *(photo 3)*. I am thinking of the most common types of lameness, in particular that which is accepted with a shrug of resignation and invariably finishes up with the pig in the knacker-cart. For instance, the case where suddenly one of a batch of sows, breeding gilts, porkers or baconers is found holding up a fore or a hind leg and looking exactly as though it has just twisted a shoulder or stifle joint.

In subacute erysipelas, the germs actually get into the joints and produce an acute inflammation when they multiply.

Chronic. This form is caused by erysipelas germs lodging in the folds of a heart valve when the bacteria are invading the bloodstream during an acute attack. What happens is that the 'bugs' multiply and grow in the valve, and eventually produce a cauliflower-like growth which is called *verrucose endocarditis*. The growth prevents the closing of the valve; blood wells back at each beat and the heart becomes enlarged and incompetent, producing what is known as an 'erysipelas heart'.

In chronic erysipelas typical symptoms appear usually after some form of stress.

3

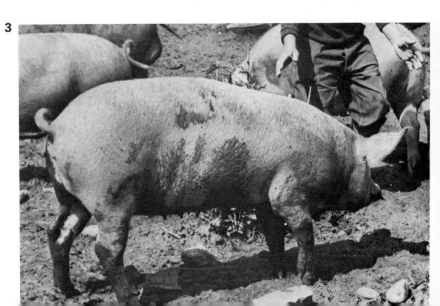

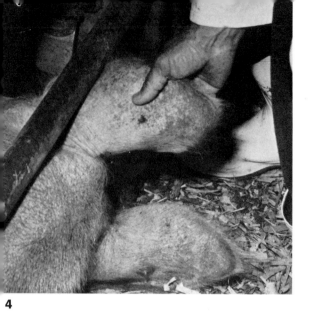

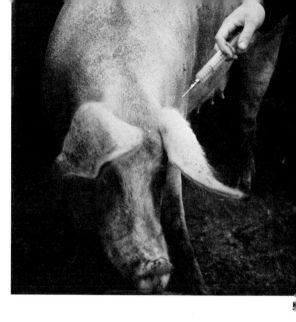

4

After farrowing or after being chased around, the pig behaves as though it has pneumonia with rapid distressed breathing. Often the ears turn blue. Occasionally after farrowing the sow may not breathe heavily but may simply go off her food. She will lie about and her ears will be ice-cold to the touch *(photo 4)*. However, if you do force her to move about, the heavy breathing and discoloration soon manifest themselves.

Treatment

In *acute cases* prompt treatment with antibiotic injections *(photo 5)* produces a spectacular recovery though it still leaves a small percentage with the chronic heart. In general, the longer you delay treatment the more likely the heart will be to develop

endocarditis. However, it never is wise to breed from a recovered case of erysipelas.

In the *subacute form* prompt treatment is also vital. A delay of even 24 hours can produce an incurable arthritis. Treatment comprises a full 5-day course of antibiotics and cortisone given intramuscularly.

Chronic swine erysipelas is incurable, though heavy doses of antibiotic may occasionally keep an affected sow going long enough to rear her piglets until they are eating solid food. If the odd sow does appear to recover completely then it is unwise to breed from her again.

Prevention

Vaccination against swine erysipelas is effective and cheap *(photo 6)*. All stock intended for breeding should be vaccinated at the age of 5 weeks and conscientiously every 6 months thereafter. I personally don't think it's necessary or economical to vaccinate stock intended for pork or bacon. The disease is never likely to become epidemic, and treatment of both the acute and subacute cases is usually successful. Also, as in so many other diseases, sound hygienic precautions will keep erysipelas among the fatteners to an absolute minimum.

Boars should be vaccinated every 6 months and if total cover is required vaccination is normally practised in recently weaned pigs (for fattener) protection and in breeding gilts or sows before service.

6

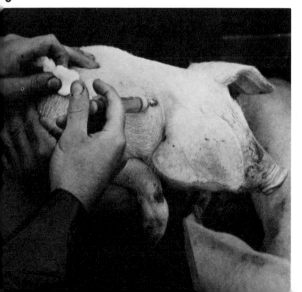

GENERAL DISEASES
AND AILMENTS

1

Notifiable Diseases

THERE are six scheduled pig diseases, that is diseases under the official control of the Animal Health Division of The Ministry of Agriculture and Fisheries.

These scheduled diseases are:

- Anthrax.
- Swine fever.
- Foot-and-mouth disease.
- Vesicular disease.
- Teschen disease.
- Aujeszky's disease.

Anthrax

Many farmers forget or don't know that anthrax can and does occasionally affect pigs *(photo 1)*.

Cause
It is caused by the same germ that produces anthrax in cattle, sheep and horses, i.e. *Bacillus anthracis*.

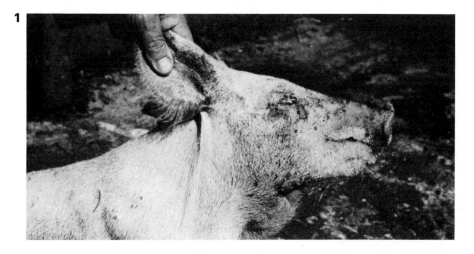

1

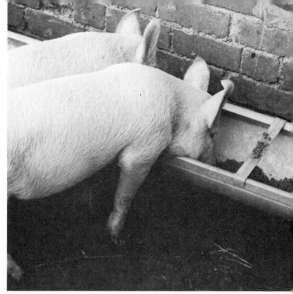

Where Does The Germ Come From?

Bacillus anthracis reaches the pig via contaminated, imported feedingstuffs *(photo 2)*. Very occasionally the odd case may arise from the eating of unboiled swill containing the flesh of affected animals.

How To Recognise Anthrax

There are two types in pigs:
1. Throat-and-neck form.
2. Abdominal type.

In the throat-and-neck type the pig goes off its feed, runs a high temperature and shows a marked swelling (oedema) under the jaw. The pig has difficulty in breathing, often snores, and white froth gathers round its mouth.

The swelling gets rapidly larger and the mechanical pressure of it at the back of the pig's throat often causes vomiting. Death usually follows, though occasionally penicillin injections can produce a cure.

In the abdominal type of anthrax the pig may just die suddenly *(photo 3)*. If it lives for a few hours it runs a temperature of up to 108° F and has bloodstained diarrhoea.

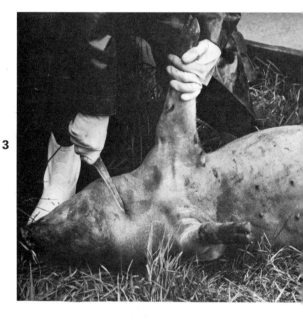

What To Do About It

In all cases of inappetance and marked swelling under the jaw and throat, or acute illness and rapid death (especially if there are signs of bloody diarrhoea), report the case immediately to your veterinary surgeon or the police *(photo 4)*. The Ministry will pay for the investigation.

A pig infected with anthrax is a source of danger to humans especially butchers and knacker men who will be the first to handle the raw carcase.

Can Anthrax Be Prevented?

There is an antiserum against anthrax but the disease is so comparatively uncommon in pigs that the routine use of antisera should never be contemplated.

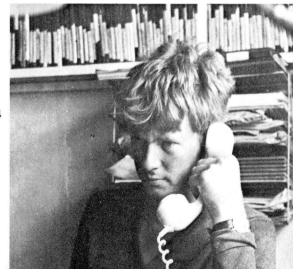

Swine Fever *(Hog Cholera)*

FORTUNATELY this virus disease has been virtually eradicated from Great Britain, but since there is a likelihood for some time at least of outbreaks of swine fever being brought into the country in imported pork or bacon I think every pig farmer should know something about it and retain a mental picture of what the disease looks like.

Clinical Picture

I regard swine fever rather like distemper in dogs in that the initial attack of the virus produces multiple small haemorrhages all over the body and it is the invasion of these damaged tissues by bacteria which produces what we recognise as the typical symptoms.

From a practical point of view I always found 'swaying on the hind legs like drunken men' is the most typical diagnostic feature *(photo 1)*. This symptom results from kidney damage. If you add to the 'drunken' symptoms a persistently high temperature which is unaffected by antibiotic treatment then it's more than likely you have swine fever.

The other typical symptoms arise from damage elsewhere—such as chronic foetid diarrhoea from an infected or ulcerated gut, coughing and pneumonia from bacterial invasion of the lung and sudden deaths from acute septicaemia.

In the early stages the first sign may be that a number of pigs refuse to eat. They huddle together, often shivering. If made to stand they may waddle with their backs arched and tails down towards the trough or drinking bowl. After that the offensive diarrhoea, the coughing and the 'drunken' stagger develop.

Perhaps the most solid practical fact that I established over many years of experience of the disease was that where persistent deaths and apparently incurable illness with varied symptoms were occurring over a period of time, swine fever was eventually diagnosed.

What To Do About It

At the slightest suspicion of swine fever or where deaths are occurring in any pig enterprise, the veterinary surgeon should always be consulted *(photo 2)*. Remember full compensation is payable.

1

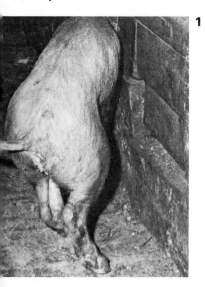

2

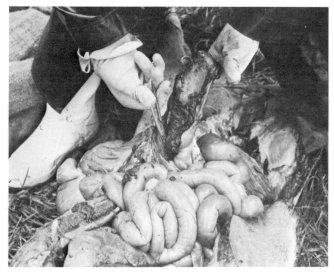

Foot-and-mouth Disease

OUTBREAKS of foot-and-mouth disease which occur in this country are due to the importation of the causal virus in infected carcases. Because of this the disease is most likely to flare up in pigs. Why?—simply because portions of the affected carcases, especially the bones, reach our pigs via the swill tub *(photo 1)*.

Clinical Picture

Initially the virus of foot-and-mouth produces a fever, and blisters or blebs may appear on the feet, snout, udder, teats and mouth. During this fever stage the pigs will be off colour and off their food, but within a couple of days the temperature drops and the pigs apparently recover.

It is then that the main observable symptom in pigs starts to appear—i.e. lameness due to secondary infection introduced when the blisters *(photo 2)* burst between the toes but especially around the coronets. Here the infection eventually causes a distinct separation of the claw.

The important thing to remember, therefore, is that primary outbreaks of foot-and-mouth disease are most likely to occur in swill-fed pigs and that lameness in any group of pigs must always be regarded as highly suspicious.

What To Do About It

Report your suspicions to your veterinary surgeon immediately.

Can Foot-and-mouth Disease Be Prevented?

If swill feeding is practised then careful and conscientious boiling according to regulations will undoubtedly kill the virus and prevent an outbreak. One of the main dangers to guard against, however, is the looting of unboiled swill either by the pigs or by dogs.

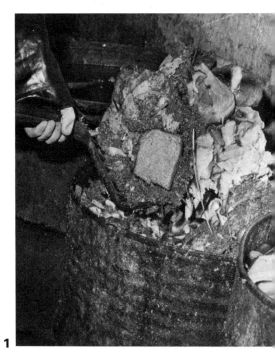

1

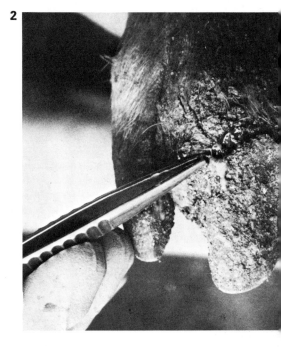

2

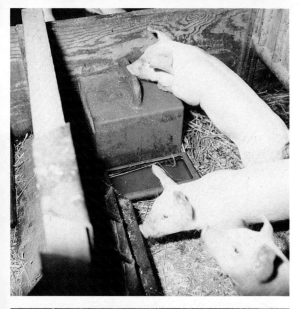

The older type of drinkers — for use with medicated drinking water (page 57).

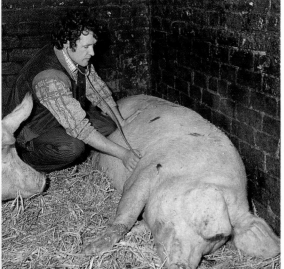

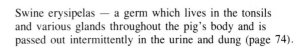

Swine erysipelas — a germ which lives in the tonsils and various glands throughout the pig's body and is passed out intermittently in the urine and dung (page 74).

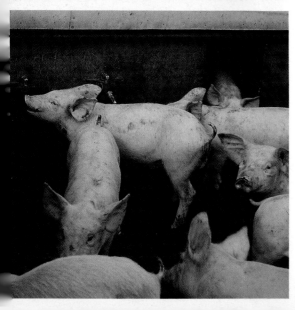

Early parakeratosis — a disease of the upper layers of skin (page 86).

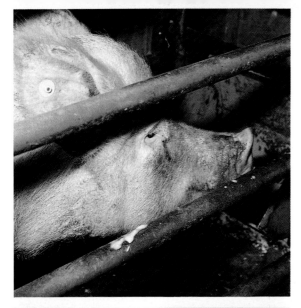

An early sarcoptic mange affecting the sow's snout (page 89).

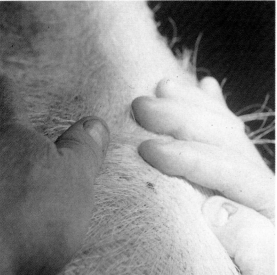

Louse infestation which is characterised by severe itching and picked up from direct contact from an infected sow or from a pen recently occupied by lousy pigs (page 94).

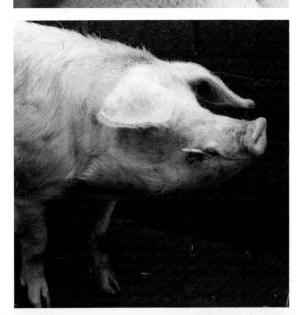

The dangerous bottom tusks of the boar which should be sawn off using "embryotomy" wire (page 151).

Vesicular Exanthema and Vesicular Disease

VESICULAR EXANTHEMA is an acute febrile infectious disease of pigs caused by a virus *(photo 1)*. It is clinically identical to foot-and-mouth. Recorded in Hawaii and the Philippines, it was eradicated from the USA in 1956, and several outbreaks occurred in Britain during the Second World War.

Recently a similar condition, called vesicular disease, probably caused by a more virulent strain of the exanthema virus, has flared up in England. Previously this strain had been reported only in Hong Kong and Italy.

Fortunately both these diseases affect only pigs so the potential danger is nothing like as great as with foot-and-mouth.

The symptoms are indistinguishable from foot-and-mouth. There is no satisfactory treatment and complete eradication must be the policy wherever practicable.

Prevention

When the disease breaks out in your area, there are certain commonsense precautions to take:

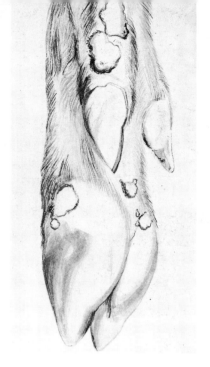

1. Keep clear of all other pig units.
2. Keep ALL strangers out of your unit.
3. Change clothes and boots before going to market and immediately on return, or – preferably – stay at home till the area is clear.
4. The source of the virus is unprocessed swill, so never be tempted to feed swill unless it has been treated as prescribed by law.
5. Report any suspect case immediately to your veterinary surgeon or to the police.

N.B. AFRICAN SWINE FEVER, which does not occur in Britain, is caused by an unrelated virus which produces similar symptoms to *Hog Cholera*. It is now seen mostly in the Iberian peninsula, Brazil and Haiti.

Teschen Disease

SO FAR this disease has not been recorded in Britain though it is listed as a notifiable disease. At present the two main countries affected are Czechoslovakia and Madagascar. Pigs of any age can be affected.

Cause and Symptoms (see page 20)

Aujeszky's Disease *(Pseudo Rabies)*

Aujeszky's disease is a herpes virus infection of pigs which causes nervous and respiratory symptoms together with a rise in temperature and often death in young pigs. In adults the only evidence of the disease may be stillbirths or abortion in the gilts or sows.

As a notifiable disease Aujeszky's disease is now being eradicated in Britain.

Cause

A herpes virus, different strains of which produce either predominant nervous or pneumonia symptoms. The virus is inhaled and gains entrance through the lining of the upper respiratory tract.

The virus is spread by 'carrier' pigs which remain infective for at least a week after recovery. The virus can also live in empty buildings for up to 6 or 7 weeks. Rats may act as reservoirs of infection.

Symptoms

Most marked in suckling pigs *(photo 1)* though I have seen the disease in recently weaned litters.

The affected piglet runs a temperature of around 105°F, goes off its feed and may or may not shiver. It then starts wandering around and falls down in a fit. If under 3 weeks old, one fit follows another until the piglet dies.

In pigs 3–10 weeks old the convulsions are irregular and seem to be triggered off by any sudden noise. The patients go off their legs, lie on their sides and paddle furiously if disturbed.

Over 10 weeks, usually in pigs 3–5 months old, there often occurs merely a 24-hour fever and no nervous symptoms develop: or the fever (105°F–107°F) may last for up to a week or longer in which case the patient stops eating, vomits occasionally during the first 3 days and shows nervous signs of trembling and staggering after the fourth day going into fits and death. Sometimes a severe pneumonia is present.

In adults no symptoms may be apparent but usually there is a rise in temperature, coughing, constipation and depression. Needless to say such cases go off their feed though many recover after 4 or 5 days.

In affected pregnant gilts and sows up to 50 per cent abort or give birth to mummified or macerated foetuses.

Control

No satisfactory treatment. Suspect cases in Britain must be reported either to the veterinary surgeon, the police or the Animal Health Division of the Ministry of Agriculture, Fisheries and Food.

Vaccination has been tried in France and eastern Europe.

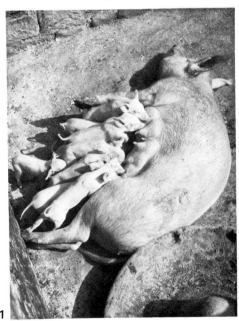

1

2
Skin Diseases

Ringworm

RINGWORM in pigs is not common; in fact it's very uncommon and yet I am so often asked about it that I think it is worth while devoting some space to it.

What Causes Ringworm?
A fungus called *Trichophyton mentagrophytes*.

What Does It Look Like?
I think the important thing to bear in mind is that the 'ringworms' look much the same as in other species, especially cattle and horses. The outbreaks occur mostly behind the ear, on the back, head and flanks *(photo 1)*.

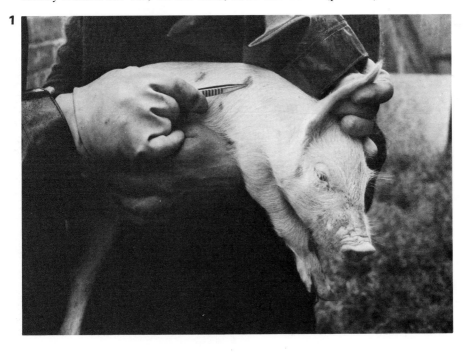

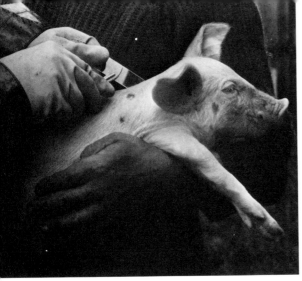

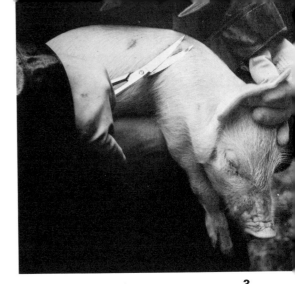

3

2

The lesions start as small, raised, greyish-coloured pustules. They become covered over with thickened reddish scabs. These then start to spread outwards in typical ringworm style, with the centres of the ringworms healing up and leaving bare dry areas.

Funnily enough some people say that ringworms on a pig don't itch. I say this is nonsense. Rubbing and irritation are part of the clinical picture.

If you want to be sure of your diagnosis, however, then it's a job for your veterinary surgeon. He will take skin scrapings *(photo 2)* and identify the spores of the fungus in the laboratory.

Treatment

Clip the hair over the area *(photo 3)* then scrub the lesions with hot water and soda.

Then apply an antifungal dressing obtained from your veterinary surgeon. In severe cases he may prescribe a course of griseofulvin in the feed.

Prevention Of Further Spread

When ringworm becomes established it will spread readily. So it is important to isolate the affected pigs not only during treatment but until the areas have completely healed.

All walls, posts and trees that the ringworm pigs have been rubbing against should be scrubbed down with hot soda

water, and either gone over with a flame-gun *(photo 4)* or painted over with tincture of iodine. Iodine has always been useful against ringworm fungus, but it is better not to use it on the pig's skin since it tends to burn the surface and either allows the fungus to spread or predisposes to secondary infection.

4

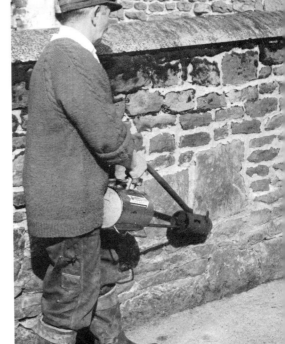

Other Fungal Conditions

Several other fungi can occasionally produce skin lesions, e.g. Candida albicans flourishes under moist conditions and fungi which grow on damp feed or grain.

However, such infections are rare and require skilled veterinary diagnosis.

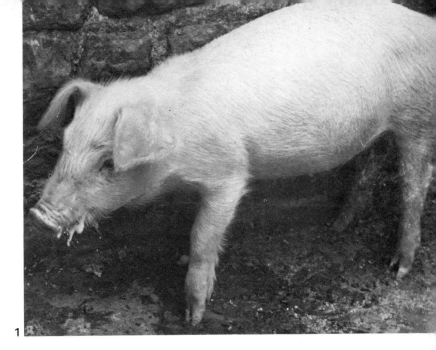

1

Pityriasis rosea

PITYRIASIS ROSEA has already been mentioned in the chapter on congenital conditions, but since pityriasis is undoubtedly on the increase in certain areas, and since it is often diagnosed as ringworm, I'd like to describe it in a little more detail.

Symptoms

Pityriasis rosea occurs only in piglets, and usually when they are 3 to 4 weeks old. It may be seen in individual piglets or the whole litter may be affected.

When it starts the piglet may go off its food, vomit *(photo 1)* and even have diarrhoea. But, as soon as the skin rash appears, these digestive disturbances disappear.

The rash breaks out chiefly on the belly of the piglet, though I've seen it cover most of the body. It starts with a number of pea-sized red spots which may join up to form larger nodules *(photo 2)*.

The spots have a crater-like surface—depressed in the centre and covered over with a brown scab. The latter comes away from the centre and the crater becomes deeper *(photo 3)*.

Needless to say the piglets lose condition.

3

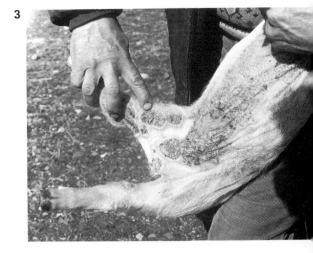

2

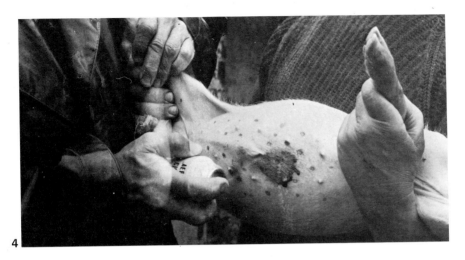

4

Treatment

The lesions heal in two or three weeks, but it as well to use a suitable antiseptic ointment or aerosol dressing *(photo 4)* under the direction of your veterinary surgeon.

Prevention

Since pityriasis is a congenital condition, the only satisfactory prevention is to change the boar and to test his successor out on the same sows.

Parakeratosis

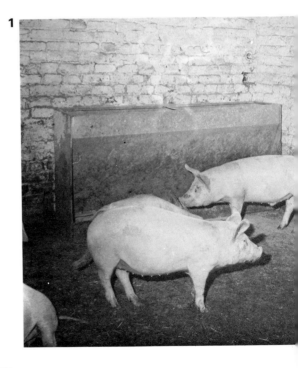

1

PARAKERATOSIS is a disease of the upper layers of the skin. It is non-inflammatory though unsightly and almost invariably gets better. It occurs most often when the pigs are dry-fed *(photo 1)*.

Cause

This is not fully established but it is known to be a metabolic disturbance associated with a deficiency of essential fatty acids. This deficiency appears to be wrapped up with the calcium:zinc ratio.

Symptoms

It starts with small pustules breaking out on the surface of the belly and thighs, though this early evidence generally goes unnoticed.

First obvious sign is usually the appearance of red spots on the legs, tail, ears, head, shoulders and flanks *(photo 2)*. These spots become raised up and covered over with hard, dry crusts. Typical lesions usually show first on the legs, especially around the knees, fetlocks and hocks.

Sometimes virtually the whole body becomes covered over with the hard, crusty areas.

As a general rule there is a minimum of rubbing and scratching, although if secondary infection is allowed to develop the pigs are far from comfortable.

They usually eat less and this plays havoc with their food conversion rate.

Only skin disease likely to be mistaken for parakeratosis is sarcoptic mange. It is best to leave the differential diagnosis to your veterinary surgeon. One outstanding difference, of course, is that mange produces severe itching right from the start whereas with parakeratosis itching and rubbing are slight.

Treatment

When parakeratosis has been diagnosed, if feeding dry, change the affected pen onto wet feeding immediately *(photo 3)* then consult the nutritional experts.

If it occurs on wet-feeding the addition of soya bean oil to the ration will produce a spectacular cure.

Prevention

The disease can be completely prevented by feeding a ration containing approximately 12 lb of calcium per ton and supplemented by a zinc salt—zinc sulphate or zinc carbonate—added at the rate of 0·02 per cent or 0·4 lb per ton.

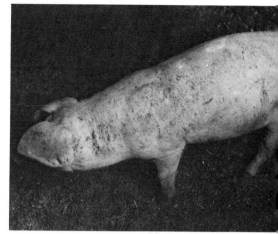

2

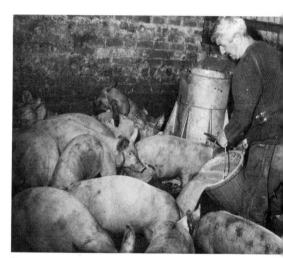

3

'Marmite' Disease

SEEN occasionally in pigs 3–6 weeks old.

Cause

Thought to be a deficiency of riboflavin.

Symptoms

Patchy reddening, with little or no itching on the ear flaps, face and abdomen. If neglected, there occurs a serous discharge and the lesions scab over. Growth is slow and there may be conjunctivitis and diarrhoea.

Treatment

Marmite on teats of sow plus multivitamin injections to piglets.

87

Pig Pox *(Swine Pox)*

THERE is one other skin disease of pigs worthy of mention and that is *pig pox*.

Cause
Two viruses, both of which are probably related to the virus that causes pox in other animals and small-pox in humans. These viruses are very strong and can live for years in discharges.

Where Do The Viruses Come From?
From carrier pigs which show no symptoms. The viruses enter locally through skin abrasions.

What Does Pig Pox Look Like?
As in the cow, it causes blisters on the skin —especially the skin of the udder and teats of the sow *(photo 1)*. These blisters burst and produce small ulcers, which can cause marked irritation during suckling.

Occasionally a more severe type of pox will break out—blisters form all over the body, rupture, and scab over to produce a condition closely resembling parakeratosis. Suckling pigs are the most susceptible.

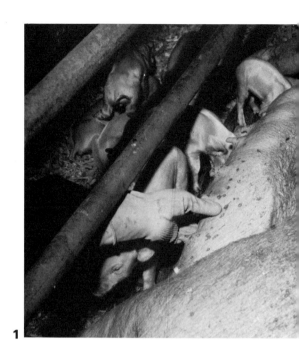

1

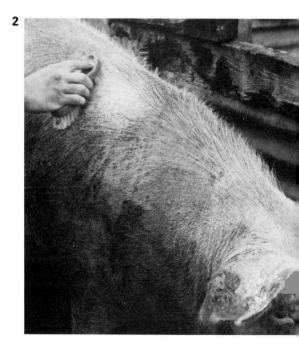

2

Treatment
Isolate the affected pig and get your veterinary surgeon to confirm the diagnosis and prescribe treatment. The patient will have to be washed in a suitable antiseptic solution containing an anti-louse agent *(photo 2)*. The pen will need to be thoroughly cleaned and disinfected, and all bedding burned.

Prevention
There is no commercial vaccine available against pox but a single attack confers a considerable degree of immunity. Control efforts, therefore, should be directed towards a correct diagnosis combined with intelligent measures to prevent spread.

3
External Parasites

THERE are only three external parasites with which we need to concern ourselves, namely sarcoptic and demodectic mange, and lice.

Sarcoptic Mange
This condition in pigs *(photo 1)* is very similar to scabies in humans.

What Causes It?
A mange parasite or mite called *Sarcoptes Scabei var suis*.

How Does It Produce Its Effect?
There are male and female mange parasites and, after mating, the female burrows into the debris in the ear or into the upper layers of the skin. In the

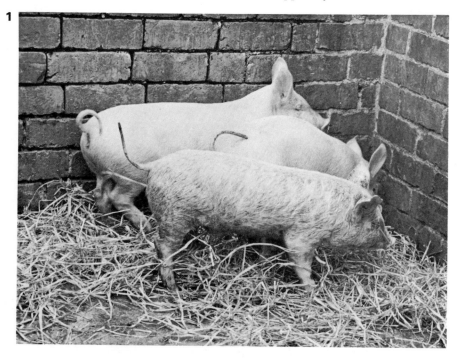
1

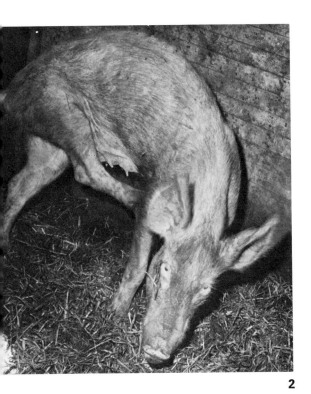

2

ticularly. Any resistance-lowering factor, like lack of milk or scours, allows the parasites to get going on the piglets.

Usually around 2 to 3 weeks the piglets start itching; the skin around the head and along the back becomes reddened, then thickened and dirty-looking. If untreated the rest of the body rapidly becomes affected and itching becomes continual. Several or all of the litter become affected and the mangy piglets soon die if not attended to promptly.

What To Do About It

First of all get your veterinary surgeon to confirm the diagnosis. He will do so by taking scrapings *(photo 3)* from inside the ear and examining them microscopically. He will then prescribe or supply a specific treatment.

It is very important to get your veterinary surgeon's advice and guidance because treatment comprises not only the destruction of all the mange mites by appropriate baths, but also the complete elimination of the resistance-lowering factors that allowed the parasites to get going in the first place, e.g. malnutrition, unsatisfactory environment, infectious disease, etc.

burrow she lays 40 to 50 eggs at regular intervals. This takes about 30 days and naturally during all the burrowing there is considerable irritation and itching. The female mite then dies but the eggs hatch out within 5 days producing 6-legged larvae which develop rapidly, through two further stages, into adults when the whole process starts again. The full cycle takes 10 to 15 days so it's easy to understand why, when mange gets a hold, the pig's condition rapidly deteriorates.

Symptoms

When the sow is badly affected she is constantly scratching *(photo 2)* and rubbing, and so quickly loses condition.

Many apparently healthy pigs, however, are carriers of the sarcoptic mange mite without ever showing any signs of the infection. These carriers are a constant menace to other younger pigs par-

3

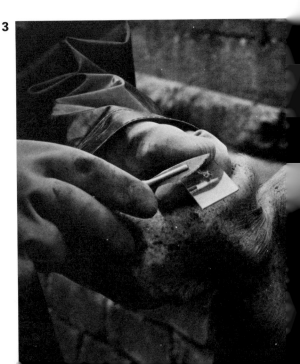

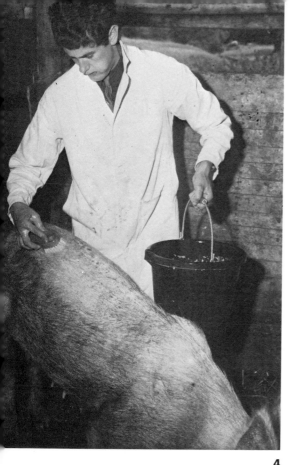

4

being brought into a clean farrowing pen.

2. All the houses, including outside yards, should be scrubbed, disinfected and gone over with a flame-gun between each batch of pigs.

3. New arrivals should be isolated and bathed three times at weekly intervals before being allowed to mix with the herd.

4. All vehicles and equipment should be treated *(photo 5)* in the same manner as the houses.

Many pig-keepers say that it is virtually impossible to eradicate sarcoptic mange because one single egg-laying parasite can produce several thousand mites within a couple of months. I know this is so, but I've found that where the job is tackled conscientiously successful eradication is attained.

I've usually found that it pays to destroy the worst affected and concentrate on the remainder, including the sow.

All should be thoroughly scrubbed with a specific mange wash *(photo 4)* once a week for 3 weeks, paying special attention to the ears, face, back and legs (thighs and armpits particularly).

Afterwards, the sow and litter should be moved to a clean, dry pen and the sow's udder wiped over before the piglets are allowed to resume sucking.

Prevention

Like all pig problems, sarcoptic mange should, if possible, be eliminated from the pig enterprise or at least rigorously controlled by commonsense preventative medicine. I recommend that:

1. Every gilt or sow should be thoroughly washed with an anti-mange preparation twice at weekly intervals before

5

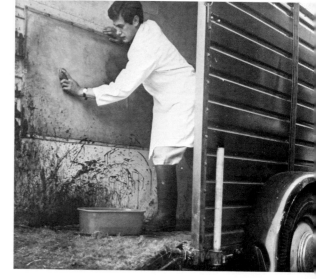

Demodectic Mange

DEMODECTIC MANGE is caused by a different type of mite called a demodex *(photo 1)*, which burrows more deeply than the sarcoptes and is consequently much more difficult to get at.

Fortunately the demodex does not spread or flare up easily and, in pigs, it rarely becomes a serious problem.

What Are The Symptoms?

An occasional piglet or older pig may show small, red, irritant dots under the neck and belly, and inside the thighs *(photo 2)*. This causes unthriftiness but usually only affects one pig in the litter. As the pig gets older the skin of the belly and thighs becomes thickened and nodules or pustules may develop.

Can Demodex Be Treated?

If your veterinary surgeon diagnoses demodectic mange he will probably not attempt to treat it. I'd say rightly so because I have never seen a case cured.

Can It Be Prevented?

It certainly can't be eradicated because of the difficulty in getting at the mite. But

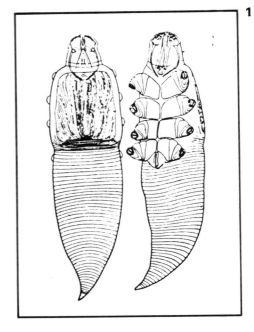

Demodex mange parasites (magnified 300 times)

demodectic mange like so many other pig conditions can be completely controlled, in my opinion, by good husbandry.

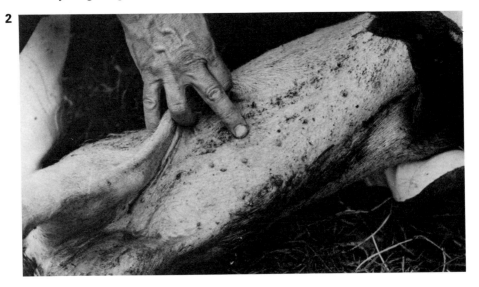

Lice

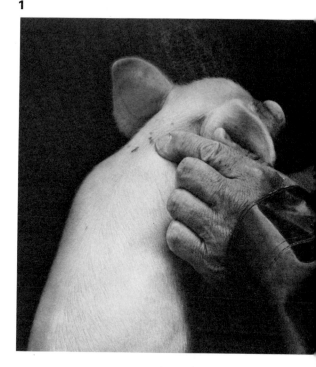

TO UNDERSTAND thoroughly louse infestation in the pig a knowledge of its life history is essential.

Life History

The pig louse is called the *Haematopinus suis*. It lives only on the pig *(photo 1)* though it can enjoy a good feed or two on man before it dies.

Again there are male and female lice; the latter lays her eggs singly, attaching them firmly at the base of the hair.

The eggs hatch out in 12–20 days, producing larvae called 'nymphs'. These then undergo three changes before becoming adult.

The adult female lays up to 90 eggs in her lifetime and starts laying about a month after she herself was an egg.

Source Of Infection

It is picked up by direct contact with an infested sow *(photo 2)* or from a dirty pen,

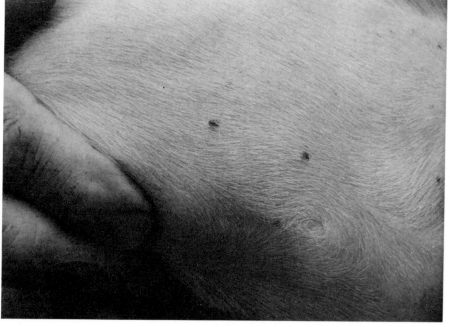

i.e. a pen recently occupied by lousy pigs.

What Is The Economic Importance
Of The Louse?

Lice puncture the skin and suck blood. This causes severe itching which makes the pig rub and scratch. Naturally a pig always on the move needs more food to take it to pork or bacon weight.

Further, lice can and do carry disease (e.g., pig pox) and the punctured wounds they produce may become infected.

Control

It is easy nowadays to treat lice, and I don't think there is any excuse at all for the presence of lice in any pig enterprise. Good housing, good husbandry and average cleanliness are all that are needed to eliminate the mites.

If you have lice on a sow and litter, then dust them both with a derris dressing *(photo 3)* once a week for 3 or 4 weeks. Among younger breeding stock three derris dressings at fortnightly intervals should see off the last of the lice.

Bought-in stock should, of course, be isolated and dressed against lice as part of the general disease prevention routine.

3

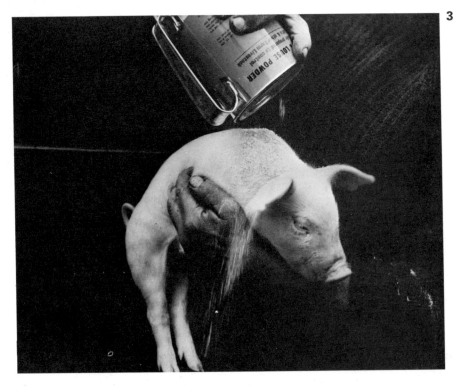

4
Worms

DURING the past few years it has been my experience that worms in pigs play a tremendously important part in the economy of any pig enterprise. Not just the large white ascarids *(photo 1)* which our forefathers have dosed against for so long, but several other parasites, which can play havoc with the pig's condition and constitution.

Worms Concerned

Ascaris—which has long been recognised —is a large white roundworm found in the small intestine.

Hyostrongylus—which lives in the stomach (mostly in sows).

Oesophagostomum (photo 2)—the nodular worm inhabiting the intestines.

Metastrongylus—the lungworm.

Trichuris—which lives in the large intestine.

Liver fluke—in grazing pigs.

Coccidia—not significant in Britain,

1

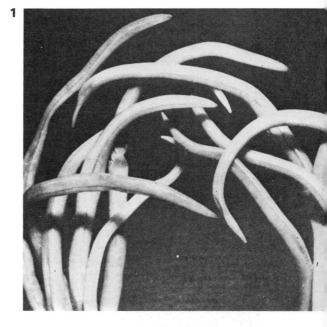

2

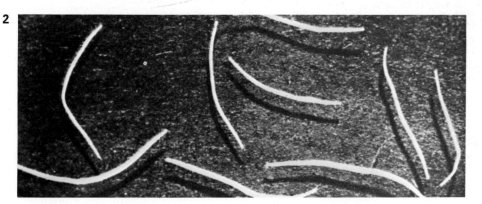

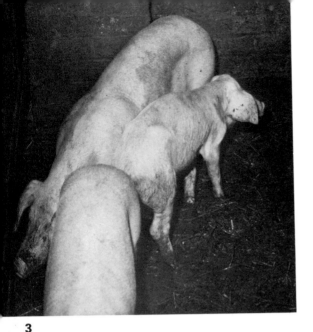

3

though they can cause diarrhoea in 5–10 day old piglets, the main source of infection being the sow.

How Do These Worms Affect the Pig?

They cause unthriftiness, poor food conversion rates and loss of condition *(photo 3)* and bodyweight. They can also lead to infertility in adult sows.

Ascaris lumbricoides during its life cycle and development passes through and damages many of the main organs of the body, especially the liver and lungs. In the liver the migrating larvae produce 'whitespot liver'. In the lungs they cause coughing and pneumonia.

Occasionally the kidneys are damaged with disastrous effects on the pig's thriftiness.

The ascaris and metastrongylus working together produce coughing which predisposes to pneumonia and general lack of condition; while the metastrongylus (the lungworm) can harbour bacteria and viruses.

The oesophagostomum causes diarrhoea and dysentery with anaemia rapidly manifesting itself, especially if the hyostrongylus is in the stomach at the same time.

The trichuris can produce diarrhoea, and it certainly retards the growth of the pig while increasing its appetite.

In adult sows, even a moderate infestation of oesophagostomum and hyostrongylus can produce infertility *(photo 4)*. The sows, especially when their resistance is low after farrowing, return to the boar and keep coming back—often irregularly. Needless to say, this can play havoc with your profits.

The hyostrongylus alone can cause the pig to eat nearly twice as much food as it would otherwise require.

What To Do

In all pig enterprises routine faecal (or dung) checks for worm eggs should be done every 6 months by your veterinary surgeon, who will then advise accordingly. The faecal samples will have to be cultured as well as examined microscopically *(photo 5)* because the oesophagostomum and

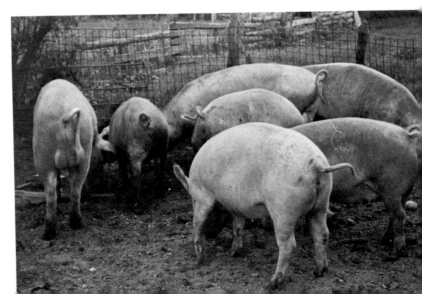

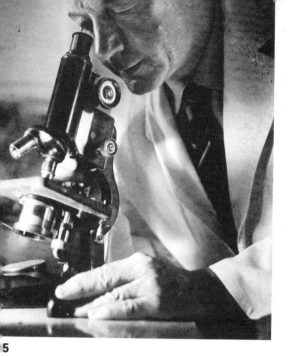

hyostrongylus eggs can only be identified after incubation.

Treatment

In a modern routine worming programme *(photo 6)* I advise treating the sows and gilts one or two weeks before farrowing, i.e. immediately before they are put into the clean farrowing pen for the first time.

Thereafter I advise dosing the young pigs at 7 weeks and again a month or 5 weeks later.

So far no single drug has been found which will destroy every type of pig worm. This is the main reason why it is essential to have veterinary advice and guidance before starting any treatment.

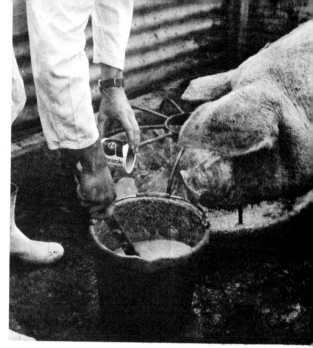

6

Prevention and Control

Under most commercial conditions control must depend on a sound routine dosing such as I have just described. But the treatment can and should be combined with sensible hygienic precautions such as:

1. After dosing housed pigs, clean and disinfect the pens *one week later*, using hot water and soda, a reputable disinfectant and plenty of elbow-grease *(photo 7)*.

2. If at pasture, move the pigs to clean ground after worming.

3. Isolate and dose all newcomers to the herd.

4. Remove all dung and bedding from the pens and hose down at least three times a week.

5. Avoid the continual use of the same paddocks for the sows and boars.

There is available a highly efficient subcutaneous injection against the ascaris, hyostrongylus and oesophagostomum. In certain circumstances the injection may be preferred to the oral dosing.

Another more advanced subcutaneous injection attacks both internal *and* external parasites (mange mites and lice). This should be used only under the supervision of a veterinary surgeon because of attendant dangers.

Highly efficient anthelmintics, which can be given in feed, are now available.

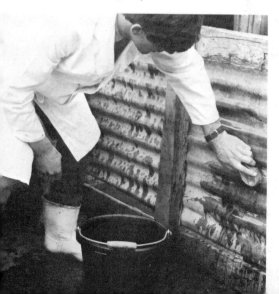

5
Deficiency Diseases

NOWADAYS, with the tremendous improvement in nutritional knowledge, deficiency diseases have largely disappeared from most pig enterprises. But when home-mixed rations or swill are being fed without the addition of reputable vitamin supplements, deficiency diseases can and do occur.

Vitamins

Vitamin A Deficiency
In gilts and sows this can cause:
- Infertility.
- The birth of dead or weak pigs *(photo 1)* with or without congenital defects like blindness and cleft palate.

In all pigs vitamin A deficiency can cause:
- Retarded growth and unthriftiness *(photo 2)* with skin changes.
- A holding of the head to one side.

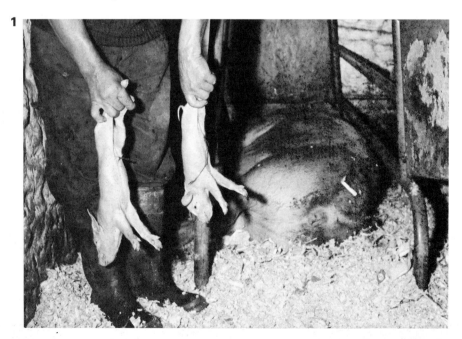

1

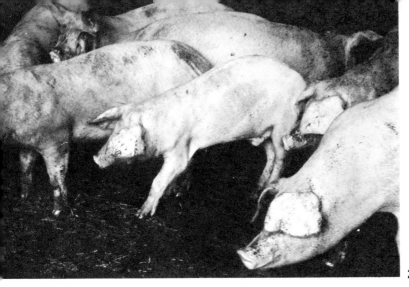

2

- Stiffness, leg weakness and eventual paralysis.
- Running eyes and blindness.

Vitamin D Deficiency

Vitamin D deficiency produces:
- Capricious appetite.
- A general unthriftiness.
- Rickets in young pigs.

Vitamin B Deficiency

Vitamin B deficiency can produce:
- Inappetance.
- Unthriftiness.
- Loss of hair and skin rashes *(photo 3)*.
- Diarrhoea and vomiting.
- Anaemia.
- Distressed breathing.

- Weakness and staggering.
- Convulsions and death.

Vitamin E Deficiency

- Muscle wasting.

This brief summary of vitamin deficiency diseases should suffice to warn all pig-keepers of the dangers of false economy in feeding.

Prevention

By all means feed swill and home-produced cereals. But for goodness sake fortify the rations with a reputable vitamin supplement *(photo 4)* and at the same time take full advantage of all the scientific nutritional advice available. There is no excuse for deficiency diseases in pigs.

4

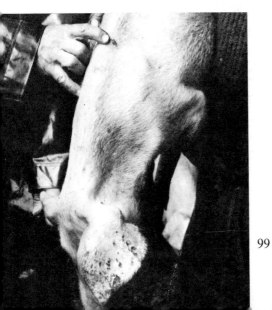

99

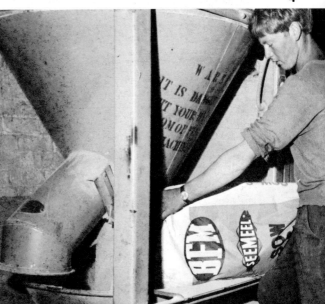

Minerals

MINERALS not only help to form the skeleton, but in combination with proteins, carbohydrates and fats, they make up many important compounds. They also play a vital part in digestion and, as soluble salts, have a wide variety of functions, including kidney filtration. In addition, they have an influence on the irritability of muscles and nerves.

Though mineral deficiencies are comparatively rare in modern pig husbandry, it is as well to keep in mind the consequences of any short-sighted economy in feeding.

Deficiency of Calcium and Phosphorus leads to rickets *(photo 1)* in young pigs and osteomalacia (brittleness in the bones) in sows.

Magnesium Deficiency can cause obscure lameness, hyper-excitability and fits.

Deficiency of Potassium, Sodium and Chlorine can trigger off digestive and kidney disorders, as well as fatigue of muscles and nerves.

Deficiency of Iron and Copper produces anaemia (see piglet anaemia), while copper shortage alone produces swayback and posterior paralysis.

Shortage of Iodine (which is essential to the correct functioning of the thyroid gland) can lead to hairless litters with thickened, pulpy skin.

Manganese is utilised in digestion and any deficiency can cause poor growth rates.

Zinc is required for the correct functioning and growth of the skin, and a deficiency produces parakeratosis (see chapter on parakeratosis).

Cobalt is another essential trace element.

It must be quite obvious that no pig enterprise can succeed unless the rations are carefully formulated by experts.

1

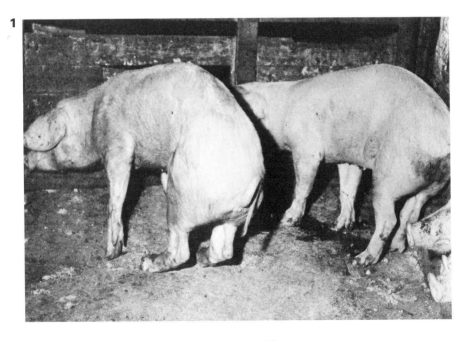

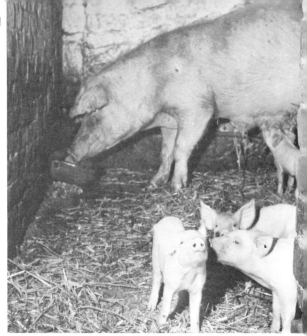

Piglet Anaemia

I WAS going to leave piglet anaemia out of the book because of the general awareness of its occurrence and the mass routine use of preventatives which now prevail everywhere.

However, certain questions fired by my latest batch of students have convinced me that the disease is well worth dealing with if only in question-and-answer form.

Piglet anaemia occurs in housed sucking pigs *(photo 1)*. It does not occur in piglets reared with access to pasture *(photo 2)*. Why?—simply because the outdoor piglet will eat grass and root in soil, both of which supply iron and traces of copper.

What Causes Anaemia?
A shortage of iron and copper in the food of the rapidly-growing piglet.

Why Not Then Feed Plenty of These Minerals To The Sow?
The sow *(photo 3)* is apparently capable of storing only a limited amount of iron,

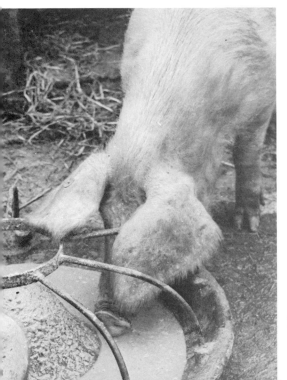

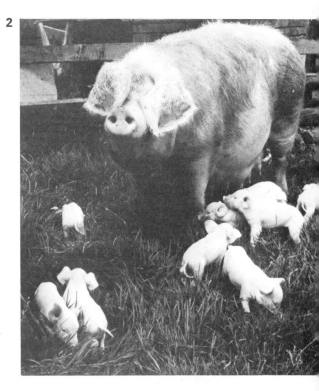

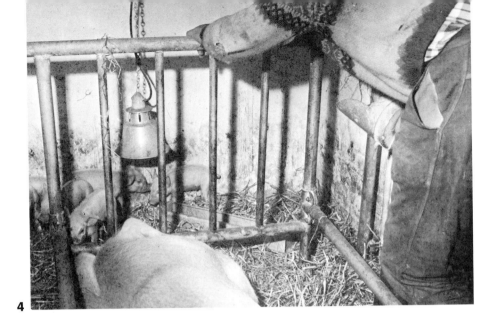

4

and the piglet's liver iron and copper reserves last only for a few days.

Can't Iron And Copper Be Provided In The Creep Feed?
Yes, but the snag is that by the time the piglets are eating sufficient creep *(photo 4)* the anaemia will probably have developed.

What Are The Clinical Signs Of Anaemia?
A yellow line along the back of the piglets associated usually, but not always, with a yellow diarrhoea *(photo 5)*.

At What Age Does Anaemia Manifest Itself?
In my experience anaemia symptoms are not apparent until the piglets are 3 weeks old.

Must Pigs Always Be Injected Against Anaemia?
Routine injections *(photo 6)* at 2 to 3 days old are essential with indoor rearing. Iron solutions or pastes (which are less expensive than the injections) can also be used and are quite efficient, but they have to be administered two or three times which means more work and more careful recording of duties.

Why Are Iron Injections So Expensive?
I don't think they are expensive and in any case one has to pay for efficiency.

5

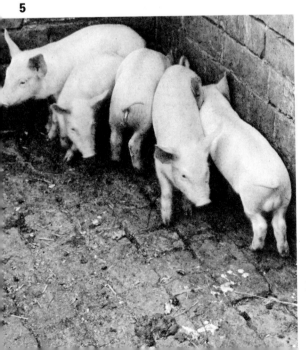

6

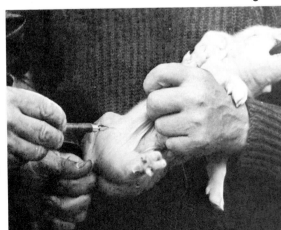

102

6
Lameness

CHIEF CAUSE of lameness *(photo 1)* in pigs, in my experience, is subacute erysipelas, or erysipeloid arthritis. But there are other bacteria which can cause arthritis and there are a number of other conditions that can produce lameness apart, of course, from joint-ill which I have already dealt with.

Infectious Arthritis

The organisms that can be involved are:
- *Erysipelothrix insidiosa.*
- *Streptococci.*
- *Staphylococci.*
- *Corynebacterium pyogenes.*
- *A mycoplasma.*
- *Haemophilus influenzae suis.*
- *E. coli.*

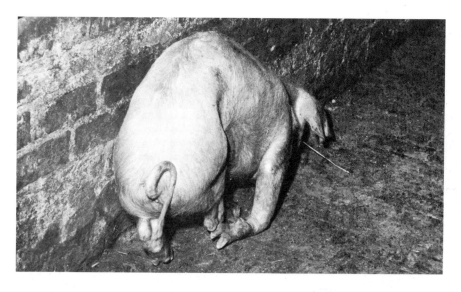

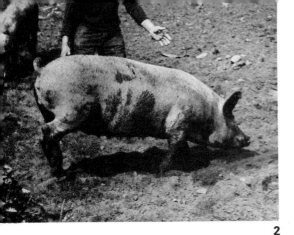

2

3

Many people have asked me if the abortion germ—*Brucella abortus*—can cause arthritis in pigs. There is so far no evidence that it does in this country, though American workers have found the *Brucella suis* involved, not only in arthritis but also in stillbirths, abortions and infertility in both sows and boars.

Clinical Picture

Sudden lameness or stiffness followed later by evidence of swelling and pain in a joint or joints *(photo 2)*.

Prevention

I have found that conscientious control of joint-ill and swine erysipelas (as advised on page 75) will reduce lameness due to arthritis to an absolute minimum in all pig enterprises.

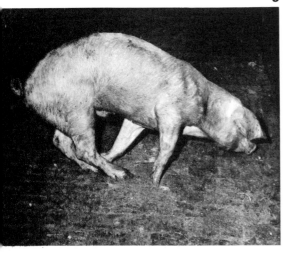

Lameness Due to Dietetical Deficiencies

Shortage of calcium, phosphorus, vitamin A, vitamin D, manganese and copper can lead to lameness *(photo 3)* and leg weakness due to changes in the actual bone structure.

Deficiency of copper, magnesium and vitamin A can lead to lameness and paralysis resulting from a damaged nervous system.

Prevention

This comprises merely making full use of all skilled advice and always carefully compounding the rations. There is no longer any excuse for deficiency lameness in pigs.

4

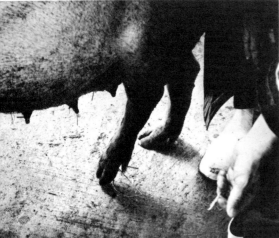

Rheumatism

Rheumatism *(photo 4)* can and does occasionally affect pigs, both as muscular rheumatism and as rheumatoid arthritis.

Cause

As in human beings, rheumatism in pigs is found where the living conditions are bad, especially where there is a cold, wet floor.

Symptoms

General stiffness and slowness in moving. When forced to move or get up the pig squeals with pain. Handling the affected muscles also causes pain.

In rheumatoid arthritis the symptoms are identical to an infectious arthritis, except that it takes longer for the joints to show external evidence of swelling and pain.

Treatment

Slaughter badly-affected pigs and treat the mild cases—after first of all making sure of the diagnosis by consulting your veterinary surgeon.

Prevention

Insulate the floors *(photo 5)* and eliminate damp and draughts from all the pens.

Apart from foot-and-mouth disease (where whole litters are likely to be lame) the other cause of lameness (and in my experience a very common cause) is some lesion of the foot or feet.

Foot Troubles

What Causes Them?

I have found that lameness in the foot *(photo 6)* is due—in order of frequency —to:

1. Mechanical injury to the foot with or without secondary abscesses.

2. Foot rot or foul in the foot *(photo 7)*, both of which are again secondary to some injury or wound and both of which involve the germ called *Fusiformis necrophorus*.

3. Continual soaking in excreta and mud which produces cracks between the claws.

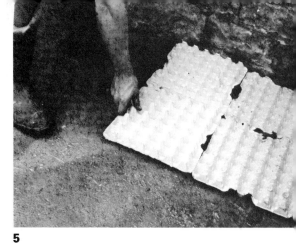

5

6

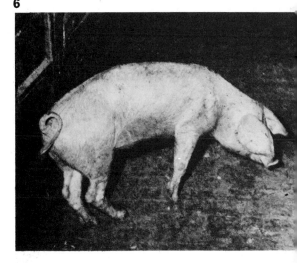

7

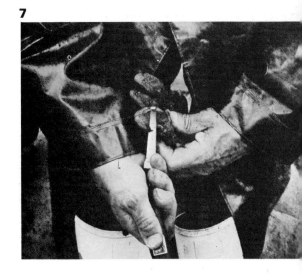

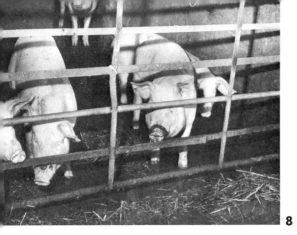

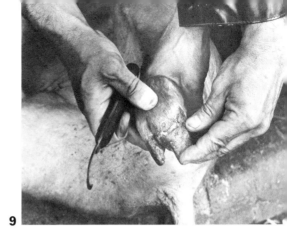

8   **9**

Often these become infected *(photo 8)*.

What To Do About It

The first and most important thing is to examine the foot thoroughly *(photo 9)* and here the pig-catcher described on page 119 will prove invaluable.

If a straightforward infected wound is found kaolin poultices should be applied and a course of antibiotics prescribed or adminstered by your veterinary surgeon.

If foot rot or foul is suspected turn the case over to your veterinary surgeon. He will remove all dead tissue, dress the wound and give the appropriate injection therapy.

How To Prevent Foot Lameness

Search around for possible causes of the mechanical injury or injuries and eliminate them. Broken or uneven surfaces at the entry or exits to pens are a likely and common cause. In fact, on the farm where this photograph *(photo 10)* was taken, foot lameness was a real headache. The trouble disappeared as soon as smooth concrete ramps were provided at the pen exits.

Dunging areas should be drained properly. Flame-gunning and scrubbing of pens are essential to keep the general bacterial population under control. But remember persistent foot lameness will never be a problem if the causes of the initial injury can be eliminated.

Sows' feet can be kept hard and healthy by providing concrete yards *(photo 11)* between the sleeping-quarters and the individual feeders.

10   **11**

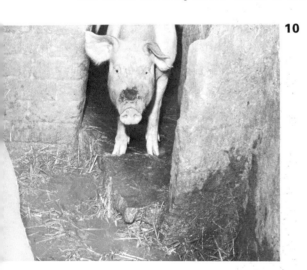

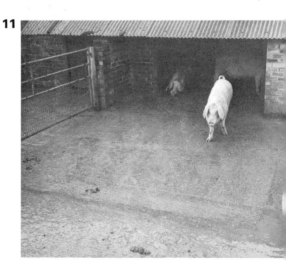

7
Vices

Tail-biting

WITHOUT doubt, tail-biting *(photo 1)* is a major headache in many pig enterprises.

Causes
Tail-biting can be triggered off by an injury to a tail. It only requires one of the pigs to start biting and the others quickly follow suit. There are, however, a

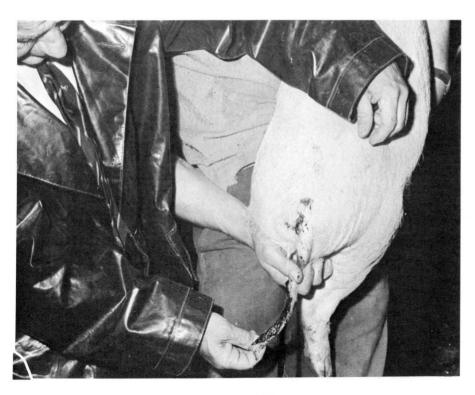

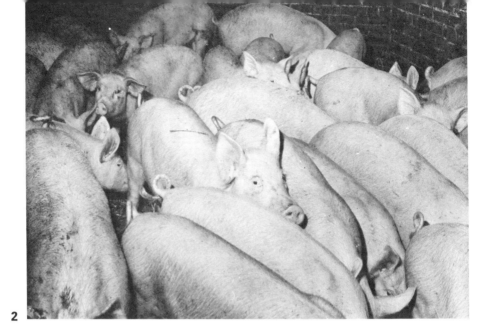

2

number of other causes which are not only much more interesting but also much more common.

The first is environment and here the main predisposing factor is excess humidity. Where you have a large number of pigs *(photo 2)* in anything like a sweat-box atmosphere, the continually-wet tail-ends may become infected with a germ called *Fusiformis necrophorus*—the same germ that causes foot rot and foul in the foot. This leads to death of the tip of the tail and the pigs immediately bite at the dead tissue.

Other environment faults which can lead to tail-biting are trapped stale air and sudden weather changes, especially in thundery weather.

3

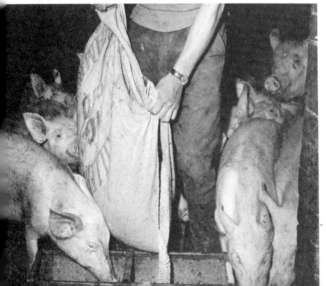

The second group of predisposing factors, and one which many people think is the most important, is found in the feeding *(photo 3)*. Certainly a straightforward shortage of protein in the diet will soon produce tail-biting but other dietetical variations have been found to trigger it off.

High-energy diets containing large proportions of wheat and maize tend to encourage it, while medium-energy rations low in animal protein can likewise be responsible. Other dietetical trigger factors?—shortage of fibre in the diet, too high or too low calcium, and deficiency of salt.

Another cause, which I have observed on a number of occasions, is a worm infestation. A pig with worms tends to swish its tail sharply and angrily. Sooner or later one of the group is attracted by the continually-moving tail and its curiosity sets off the biting sequence once more.

In fact, anything which makes the pigs restless or discontented is likely to cause trouble. And it needn't be so obvious as a swishing tail. For example, with floor-feeding *(photo 4)* and self-feeders, simple quarrelling is often caused by pigs on the move tramping on their sleeping mates. Other causes are excess dust, overcrowding, and boredom. Overcrowding by itself is not enough to start tail-biting; it only

108

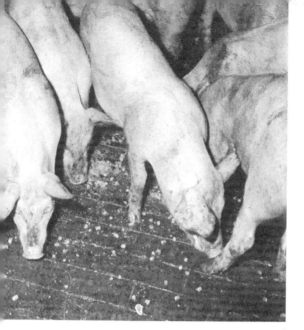

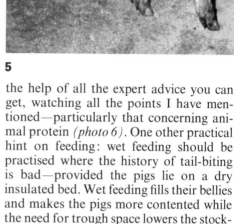

4 5

becomes important when combined with environmental or feeding faults.

One last trigger factor which occurs occasionally—puberty *(photo 5)*. I've seen tail-biting in a batch of young gilts penned up together in the spring and I'm convinced the cause was early sexual development.

Prevention And Control

Secret of prevention obviously must lie in finding the cause and rectifying it.

Here, at a glance, is a straightforward list of my hints for controlling tail-biting:

1. Eliminate excess humidity and stale air by improving the ventilation. This must be done gradually because it is just as important to maintain a constant temperature in the house. Keep the temperature at 70° F for weaners and gradually drop down to 60° F as the pigs mature to pork and bacon. Guard against rapid change by providing adequate insulation.

If relying on natural ventilation try to get the air outlet space adjusted to about 10 square inches per fattening pig, but site the outlet to prevent draught.

With power ventilation the ideal to aim at is 25 cubic feet air change per minute per 100 lb of liveweight housed; and a relative humidity of around 50 to 70 per cent.

2. Devise your rations carefully with

the help of all the expert advice you can get, watching all the points I have mentioned—particularly that concerning animal protein *(photo 6)*. One other practical hint on feeding: wet feeding should be practised where the history of tail-biting is bad—provided the pigs lie on a dry insulated bed. Wet feeding fills their bellies and makes the pigs more contented while the need for trough space lowers the stocking rate and improves the environment.

3. If worms are present make sure that routine dosing becomes an integral part of the general management (see chapter on stomach and bowel worms).

6

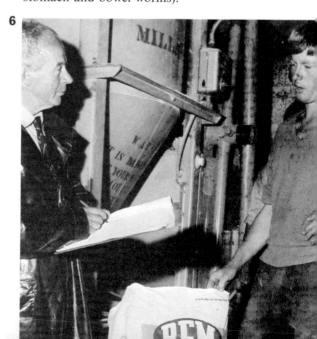

4. Alleviate boredom by any means you can think of and don't be ashamed or self-conscious if the methods you employ seem a bit outlandish to your friends. Chains *(photo 7)* hanging from the roof to the floor are as good as anything but even the simple things—like some straw *(photo 8)* twice a day, a cabbage or two, or an armful of cut grass—all help. Another useful hint is a radio kept on from early morning until last thing at night.

5. With batches of gilts in the spring—cover or darken the windows. This reduction of light seems to work in exactly the same way as it does in helping to deter feather-picking in poultry.

These then are my rules for preventing tail-biting: stick to them and the trouble will nearly always disappear. What about docking? To my mind this is a crazy waste of time and a cruel practice. The stumps will still be gnawed if any of the other pre-disposing factors are allowed to remain.

Routine tail docking, which is still practised fairly intensively, is only apparently successful because the main predisposing causes have been eliminated.

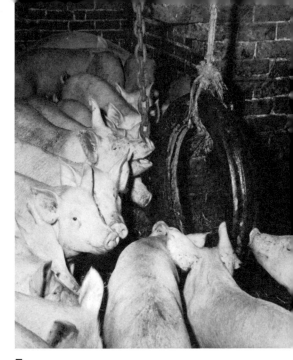

7

8

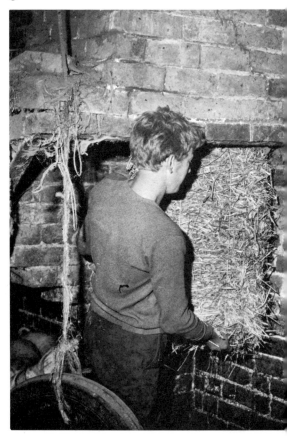

110

Ear-nibbling

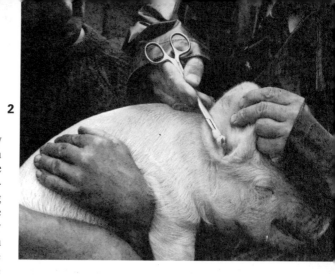

EAR-NIBBLING is almost invariably started by mange mites (see chapter on mange). What happens is that the mange mites, if untreated, produce a smelly discharge *(photo 1)* or else the mangy pig rubs the ear raw in an attempt to alleviate the itching. Fellow-pigs are attracted by the smell or the blood and the ear soon becomes a mess. The nibbled ears become infected and often the victims have to be slaughtered.

Prevention

Simply incorporate into the general routine the precautions I have outlined for mange *(photos 2 and 3)*.

Treatment

Most effective treatment I've found is to set about the pigs with a thorough course of mange baths and change the pens after each bath. Better still, if the weather allows, let the pigs run out in paddocks *(photo 4)* where they can get away from each other and give the wounds a chance to heal.

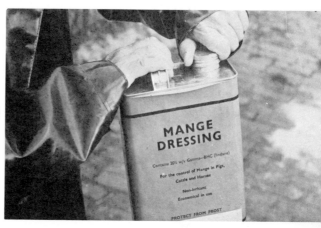

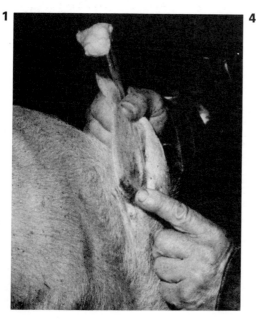

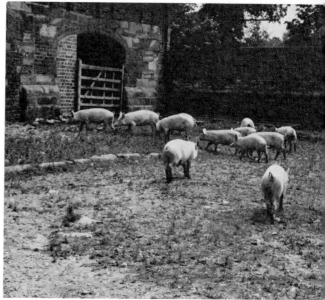

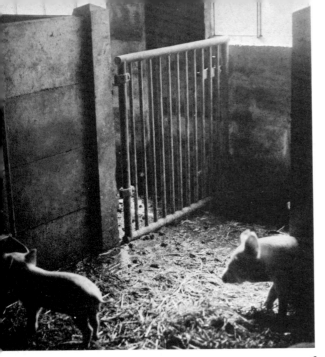

1

Soiled Bedding

SOILED BEDDING *(photo 1)* can be caused by:
- No definite division between the bed and the dunging area.
- Pigs drinking a lot of water.
- Swill feeding.
- Wet-meal feeding.
- Piped whey.
- Draught and cold in the dunging area.
- Light (especially natural light) in the sleeping-quarters.

Prevention
Once again, preventing this vice depends on eliminating the causes *(photo 2)*:
- A heavy railway-sleeper or a strong board, fixed into the floor along the front of the sleeping portion is a simple, effective, and inexpensive way of isolating the sleeping-quarters *(photo 3)*.
- The fluid intake problem is not so easily solved, particularly where pipeline feeding is practised.
- Draughts in the dunging area can be eradicated by a little ingenuity.
- The light factor can be taken care of by blanking off any windows or openings looking into the sleeping-quarters *(photo 4)*. This is perhaps the simplest but most important of all the preventative measures.

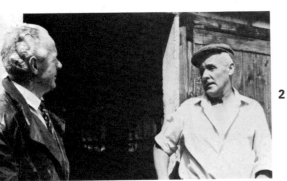

2

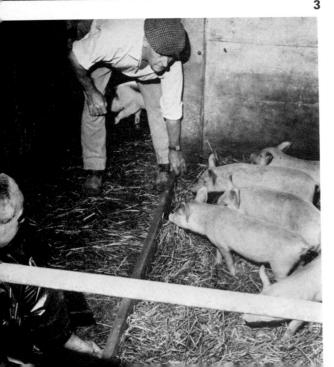

3

4

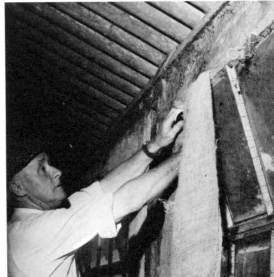

Savaging

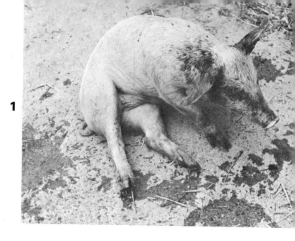

MOST OBVIOUS and common cause of savaging *(photo 1)* is the adding of new pigs to an existing pen. However, I have often seen it break out for no apparent reason in an established pen, and in such cases the cause is bullying.

If the pigs are overcrowded on a cold concrete floor then naturally they may soon start fighting for the best places to lie.

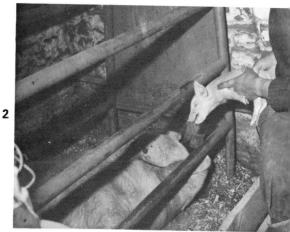

Another form of savaging occurs during farrowing *(photo 2)* when the mother may attack and kill her piglets. In a gilt this is most likely due to the pain and strangeness of her labour, although it may be an hereditary defect.

In sows, I think, bad management is often the main cause. The sow may be brought in from outside immediately before farrowing and shut in an unfamiliar farrowing pen, full of strange atmosphere and noises.

She may also object to someone sitting watching her farrow.

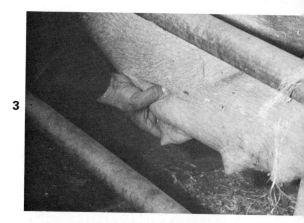

One other possible cause in both gilts and the sows is an acutely painful mastitis *(photo 3)* which may make them snap at their piglets as they attempt to suck.

How To Prevent Savaging

The golden rule again is to spot the cause and then eliminate it.

The addition of new pigs to the pen, overcrowding and cold damp floors, inadequate time to allow a sow to accustom herself to the farrowing quarters, the diagnosis of the mastitis—all these need only a little common sense and observation.

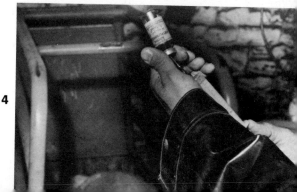

Sedatives can be given to the gilt or sow *(photo 4)*. Some people prescribe half a gallon of old ale but I usually advise fattening a gilt if she savages her first litter. I have found that if a gilt is not a good mother with the first litter she is not much better with subsequent ones. Nonetheless, 5–6 cc of the tranquilliser acetylpromazine will often see the sow over the danger period and save the litter.

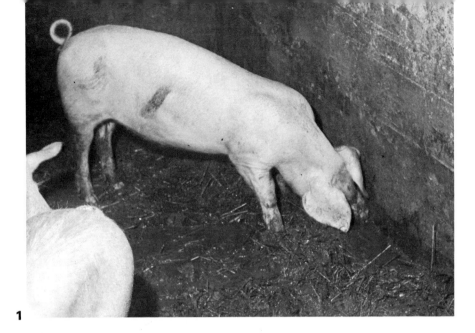

1

Depraved Appetite

HERE the vice squad eat bedding or dung, drink urine *(photo 1)* and gnaw doors and walls.

Cause
Due undoubtedly to a straightforward digestive disorder and very often associated with a lack of minerals.

Treatment
First of all treat the pigs with a laxative and then add calcium, a pinch of salt or fish meal to the food. I have always found the addition of 5–10 per cent of fish meal to be the most satisfactory cure.

Prevention
Check the rations carefully, taking full advantage of all the expert advice you can get, and always bear in mind the need for a percentage of animal protein *(photo 2)*.

2

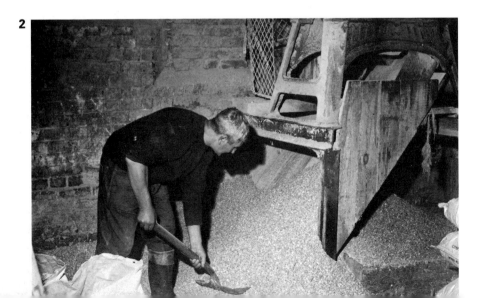

8
Sunstroke and Heat-stroke

SUNSTROKE occurs only in pigs exposed to direct sunshine, so it is seen only in outdoor pigs or in those with open exercising yards *(photo 1)*. It affects the younger pigs particularly.

Symptoms

The sun-burned pigs are reluctant to move *(photo 2)* and when forced to do so they dip in the back and go off their hind legs for a second or two. They will do this about every 30 seconds or so. If several are affected simultaneously the condition can cause real panic.

In very severe cases the pigs develop heat-stroke due apparently to the pigs' heat-regulating mechanism going haywire. Temperatures go up to a fantastic 110° or 111°F which makes the pigs stagger and shiver, salivate and breathe with difficulty.

If untreated they become frenzied, flop down, turn blue (i.e. cyanotic) and die.

Treatment

As soon as the condition has been diagnosed (and the symptoms are absolutely characteristic) the pigs should be moved

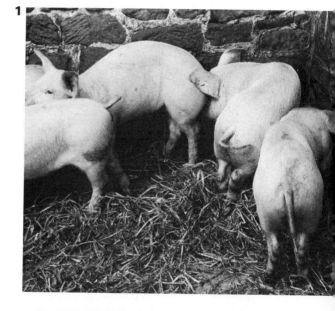

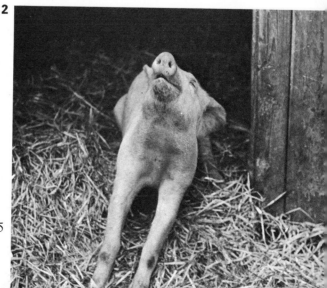

115

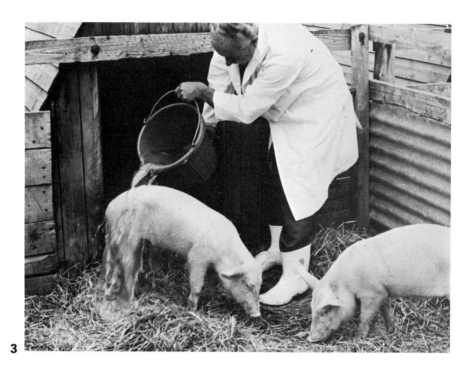

3

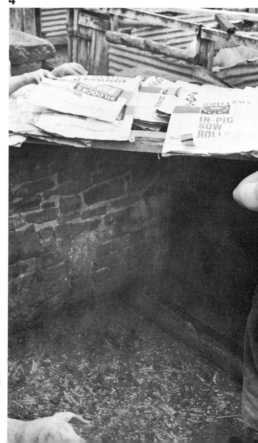

4

to a cool, dark house. Cooling lotions or anti-blister ointments can be applied to the ears and back, and antihistamine injections given against shock. Fortunately, in the vast majority of cases, the symptoms soon wear off and the pigs make a complete recovery.

If the high temperature of heat-stroke is present, then spray or drench the pigs with cold water *(photo 3)* and continue until the temperature begins to fall. If the temperature doesn't drop within an hour then emergency slaughter should be resorted to.

Prevention

This is just common sense. Shelter against direct sunshine *(photo 4)* should always be provided, especially for the younger pigs under 13 or 14 weeks of age.

In hot countries not only should there be adequate ventilation but cold running water may be needed in each pen.

116

9
Haematoma in Ear

A HAEMATOMA is a collection of blood forming a swelling. When this occurs between the layers of skin in a pig's ear *(photo 1)* it is usually caused by the pig rubbing the ear, scratching it, or shaking its head; though it can result from fighting. The pig holds its head to one side, and the obvious pain and discomfort interfere with growth rate.

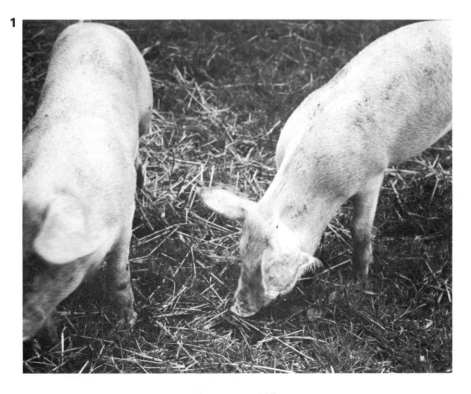

2

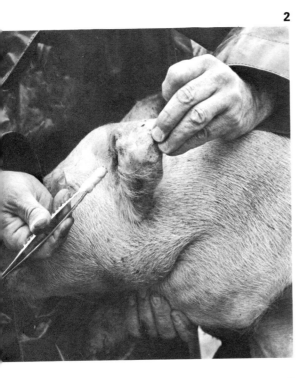

Treatment And Prevention

Usual cause of ear-rubbing is mange mites inside the ear *(photo 2)*. See chapter on mange.

The swollen ear will probably have to be operated on by your veterinary surgeon. He will open up the haematoma under local anaesthesia *(photos 3 and 4)*, curette the lining to prevent a recurrence, then suture to control haemorrhage and ensure correct drainage.

Obviously it is much better not to have to deal with this condition and the routine control of sarcoptic mange will virtually eliminate ear haematoma from the herd.

One thing is certain, this apparently simple operation should never be attempted by the pigman. If it is, then he can expect a squealing blood-bath!

3

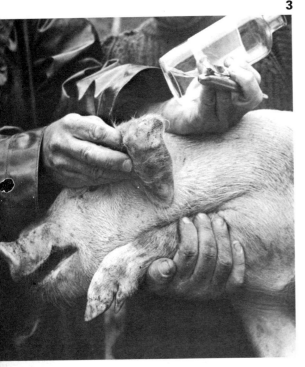

4

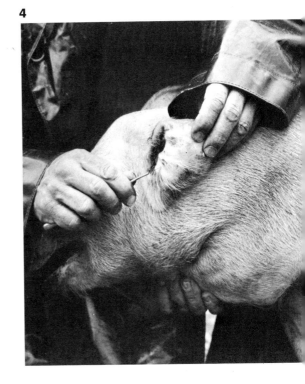

10
Prolapsed Anus and/or Rectum

PROLAPSED ANUS AND/OR RECTUM is occasionally seen in sows and it is usually caused by excessive straining during labour.

In my experience, however, it most frequently occurs among weaners or fatteners.

Cause
Too much fibre in the diet. Because of this prolapses are most likely when the rations are home-mixed. Infectious and parasitic enteritis can also predispose to prolapse.

Treatment
Never attempt to replace a prolapse. Quite apart from the pain and shock produced it will rarely stay in position even with correct anal purse-string suture. The affected pig should be isolated to prevent cannibalism. *The best treatment of all is to leave it alone.* By all means dress daily by puffing a sulpha or antibiotic powder over the mass but *never attempt to handle it*.

What happens is that within a few hours of prolapsing the blood supply is cut off by ring pressure—just as if you had tied a tight ligature around its base. All pain and sensation quickly disappear. The prolapse dies and drops off in a week or ten days.

Every one of the last fifty cases I have seen made a complete recovery without a single complication or death.

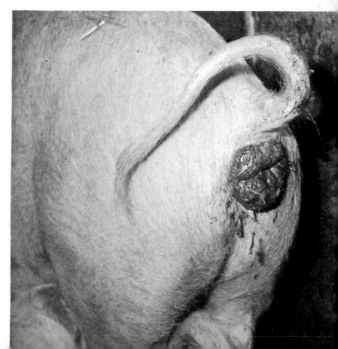

Prevention
When prolapses are occurring the fault lies in the diet, so consult your nutritional adviser immediately.

Vaginal and/or Uterine Prolapse
Vaginal prolapse is often due to tethering heavily pregnant sows with the hind-quarters lower than the body. Uterine prolapse may follow a prolonged or difficult farrowing. Both are serious and require URGENT veterinary attention.

GENERAL HINTS

1
Catching and Penning

A CATCHING CRATE is a simple piece of equipment I would recommend to every pig-keeper in the country. It will save countless hours of work and frustration. In fact it makes the handling of pigs, large and small, for castrating, marking, vaccination, etc., almost a pleasure.

It can be constructed in a few hours by any handyman. It can be any size *(photo 1)* but I've found that one big enough to take a sow is still sufficiently portable and efficient for pigs of all sizes.

It is made of light timber bolted into the lightest of angle-iron, the idea being

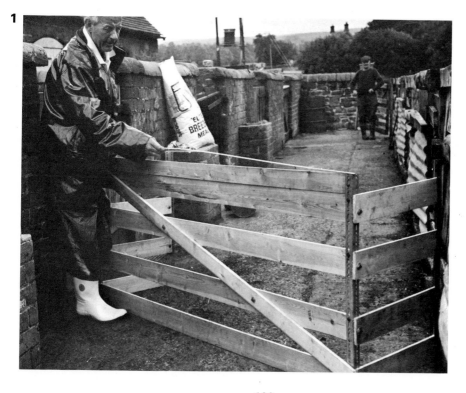

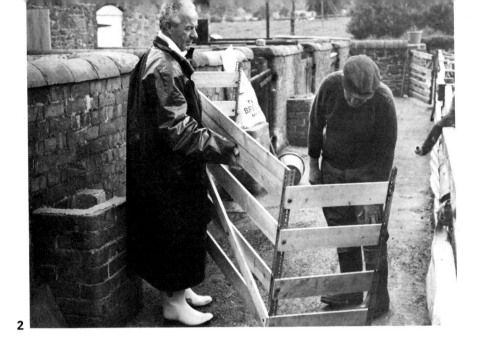

2

that one man should be able to lift it and move it around quite comfortably *(photo 2)*.

Overall length is 6 feet *(photo 3)*. This provides ample space for any sow and for most younger boars, too.

Height *(photo 4)* is 2 feet 10 inches and the spaces between the bolted timber should never exceed 4 inches. Double board at the top allows the pen to be used upside down for baby piglets. This particular crate was unfinished and required

3

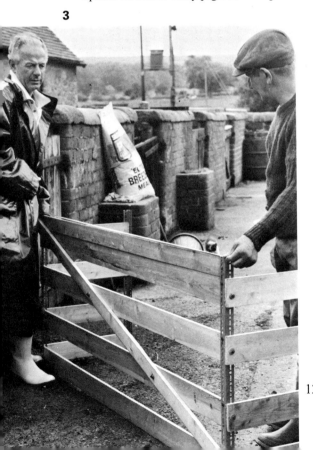

4

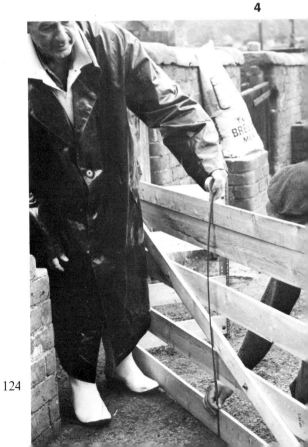

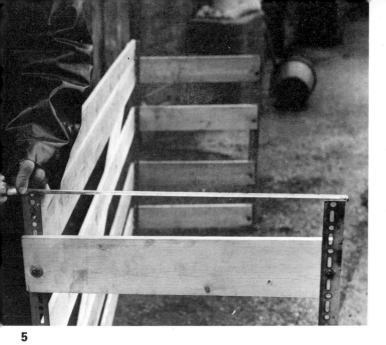

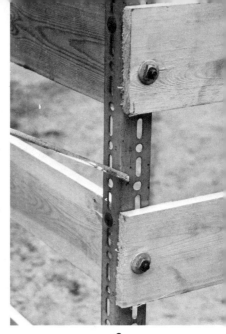

5   **6**

a continuation of the double board on both wings. It was deliberately left unfinished to illustrate the point.

Width of the wings—approximately 1 foot 9 inches *(photo 5)*; again the spaces betwen the wing timbers no more than 4 inches.

Method of fixing the timbers to the metal corner-piece is simple *(photo 6)*.

Wing timbers are bolted at both ends to the light Meccano-type angle-iron *(photo 7)*.

7

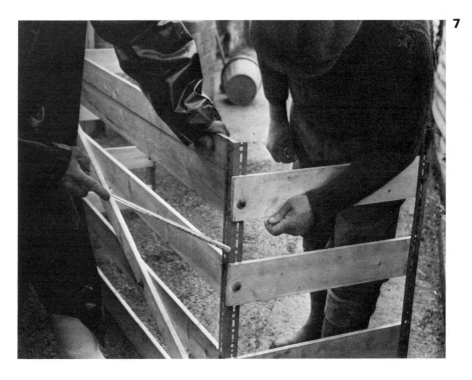

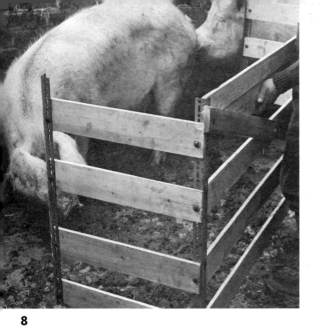

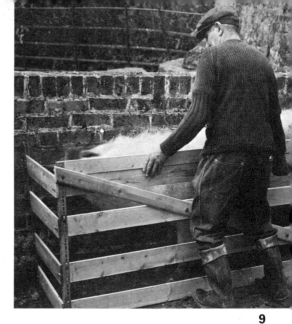

8

9

Isolating a sow for examination or injection is easy with the catching crate. Approach the sow quietly and head her towards a wall *(photo 8)*.

Clap the ends of the pen wings against the wall *(photo 9)* and you've got her. The sow will make no effort to break or jump out of the crate. Why?—simply because she can see through the spaces. If you try the same technique using solid metal or wood the sow will jump up or wrench the crate out of your hands.

Routine examination *(photo 10)* is now very simple, as is also foot examination, dressing wounds, vaccination, etc.

10

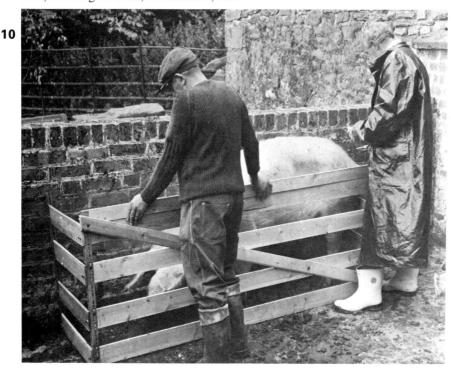

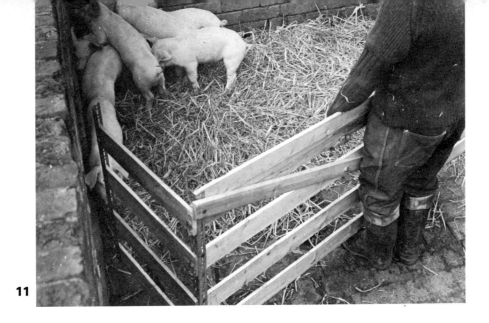

11

For catching younger pigs the identical technique is used—walk them quietly towards a wall *(photo 11)*.

When in position *(photo 12)* the crate is a god-send for injecting, vaccinating, weighing, castrating—in fact, for any routine handling job.

A similar crate made of light tubular alloy welded at the corners will last longer and will be just as portable.

The base and sides can be protected by wire mesh (see page 140).

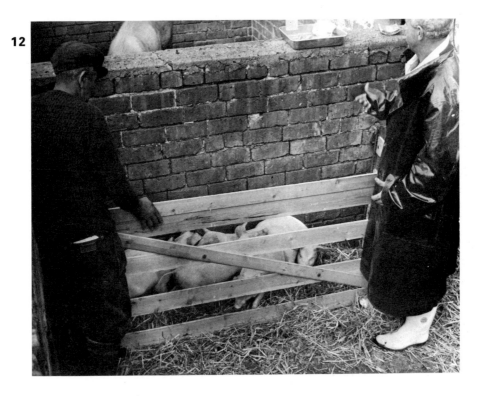

12

2
Pigman's Veterinary Kit

DISEASE CONTROL is a team job and it would become uneconomical if the veterinary surgeon had to visit and dispense every preventative inoculation. It is vital therefore that a responsible pigman should be properly equipped.

Here is the kit I recommend to all head pigmen. It should contain three syringes, a variety of needles, cotton-wool, antiseptic and sterilisation equipment *(photo 1)*.

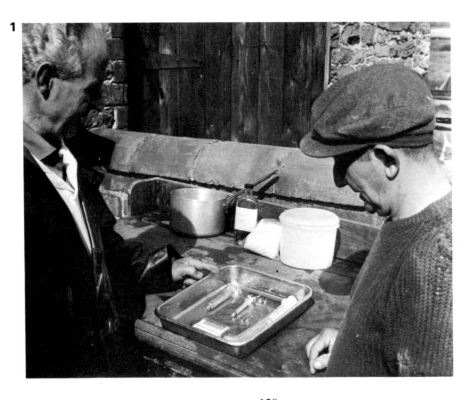

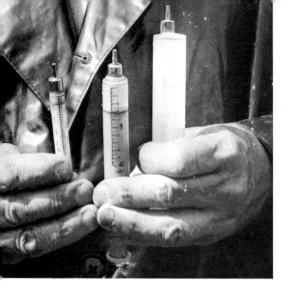
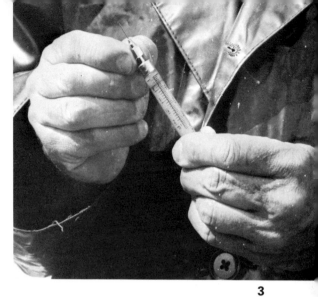

3

I prefer nylon syringes with stainless steel nozzles and I recommend a 2-cc, 10-cc and 20-cc size *(photo 2)*.

The needles must be sharp and strong *(photo 3)* and of best-quality stainless steel. This small 2-cc syringe is ideal for iron and other injections *(photo 4)* in baby piglets; the needle should be strong and fine but no longer than $\frac{1}{2}$ inch.

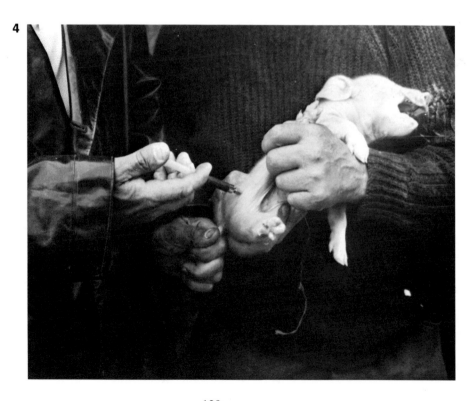

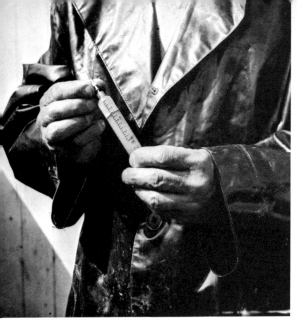

5

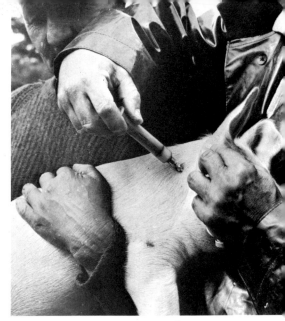

6

The larger 10-cc syringe *(photo 5)* and much stronger No. 15 ½-inch needle are admirable for use in pigs 3 weeks and older. This short, strong, ½-inch stainless steel needle *(photo 6)* will never break and will last for a long time.

The 20-cc syringe and the longer No. 15, 1-inch, stainless needle *(photo 7)* are ideal for intramuscular injections in sows and boars.

The best way of all to sterilise—boil the syringes and needles at least once a

7

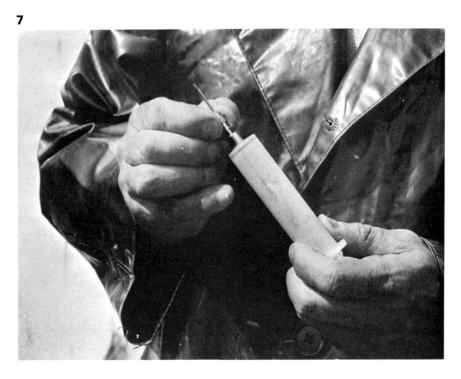

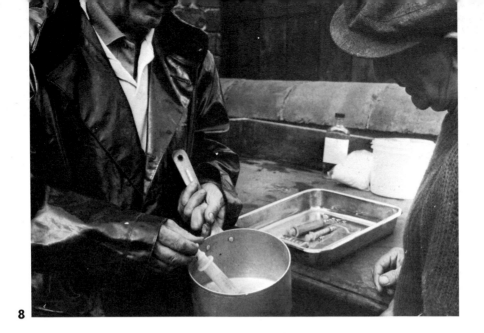

8

week in a saucepan *(photo 8)*.

For day-to-day sterilisation (which in itself is extremely efficient) a water-tight plastic container and a reputable instrument antiseptic *(photos 9 and 10)* is ideal. I always advise both, i.e. boiling once a week and constant immersion, when not in use, in the cold instrument antiseptic.

9

10

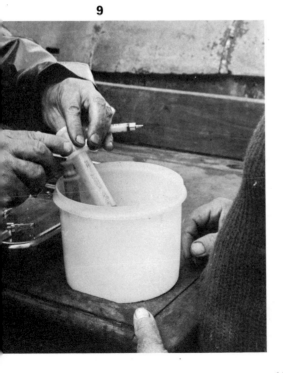

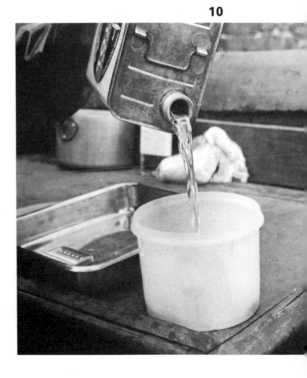

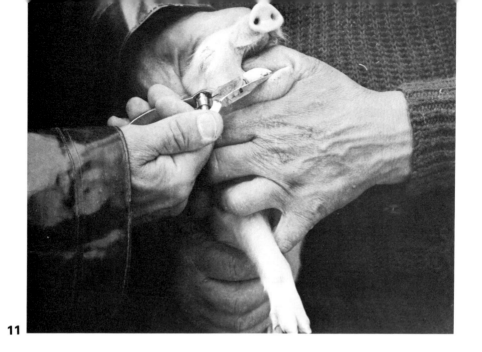

11

The only other instruments required for routine use are tooth clippers *(photo 11)* and a scalpel and a sharp blade *(photo 12)*; again these should be stored in instrument antiseptic.

12

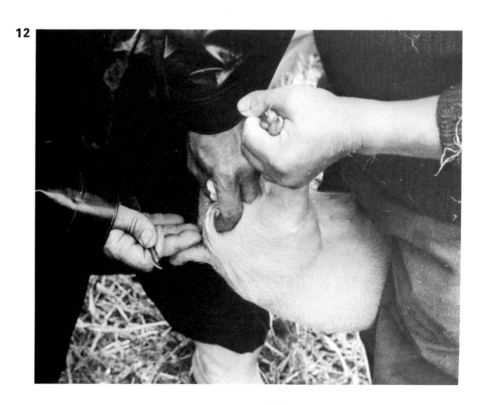

3

Injections

FOR ALL INJECTIONS *(photo 1)*, except the iron given to baby piglets, I've always found the most satisfactory site is about 1 inch behind the base of the ear. It is easy to get at and if the pig struggles the needle is not likely to break. Whenever possible the stockman should hold the pig in his arms. Injections given to the free-moving pig are never satisfactory.

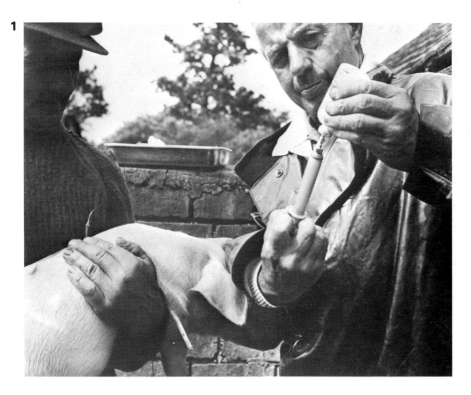

1

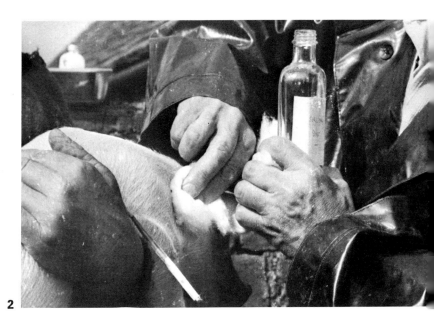

2

First swab the site with cotton-wool impregnated with surgical spirit or other skin antiseptic *(photo 2)*.

Select the site in the slight hollow approximately 1 inch from the ear base *(photo 3)*. Never go too near the ear or the injection may land in the ear cavity instead of in the muscle.

3

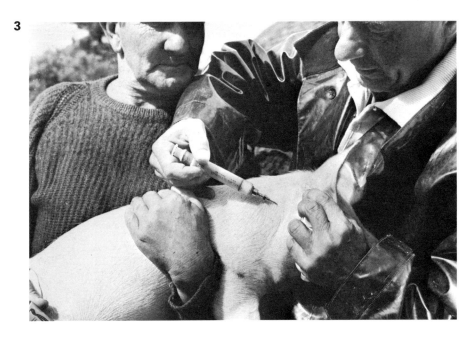

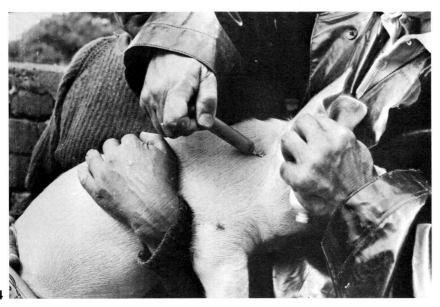

4

Don't be afraid—stick the needle straight in to its full extent perpendicularly. With the $\frac{1}{2}$-inch needle especially there is no danger of hitting the bone. Inject the syringe contents slowly and there will be little reaction *(photo 4)*.

Massage the site of the injection for just a couple of seconds *(photo 5)*. This closes up the needle hole and finishes the job off professionally.

Mark the pig *(photo 6)* and you are ready for the next.

5

6

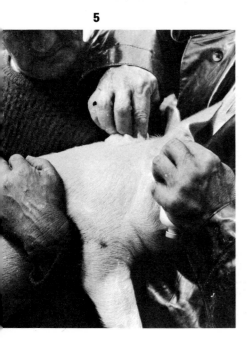

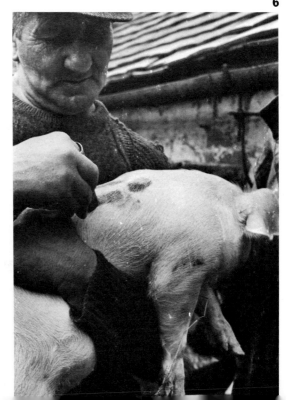

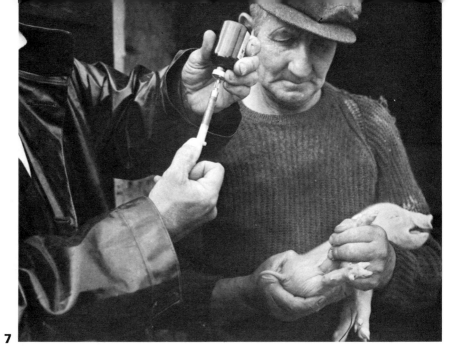

7

Research workers have found that the most satisfactory site for iron injections in the baby pig is the soft muscle at the back of the hind leg. Have the piglet held so that the chosen muscle is relaxed *(photo 7)*.

Once more select and swab the site with cotton-wool soaked in spirit or skin antiseptic *(photo 8)*.

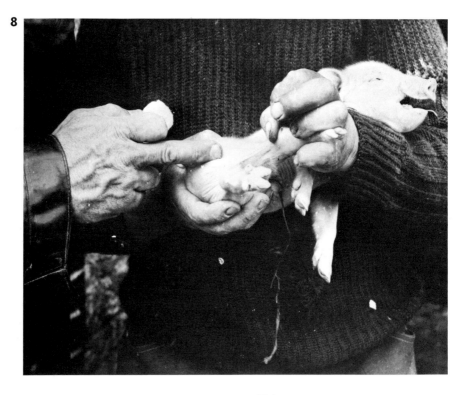

8

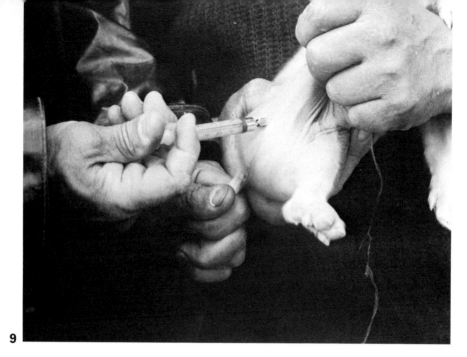

9

Stick the needle right into the belly of the muscle *(photo 9)*—it will take the full ½-inch length comfortably, and again inject very slowly. The hand holding the leg will prevent struggling which might cause a broken needle.

Finally don't forget to massage the site for a couple of seconds after the injection *(photo 10)*.

10

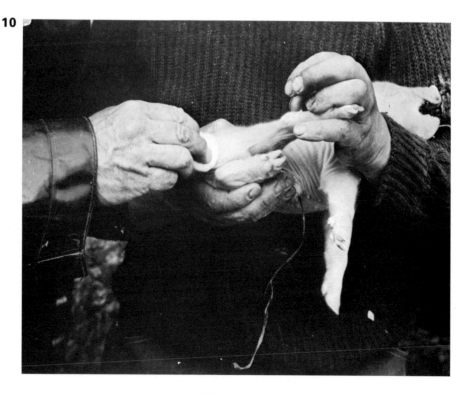

4
Castration

THERE IS now ample evidence throughout Britain, Denmark and America that the castration of a pig intended for pork is no longer necessary. Uncastrated hogs have been shown to grow better and kill out better than the castrates, and—even more important—no trace of carcase taint can be detected at slaughter.

Obviously, therefore, the time is ripe for a change in the present pig subsidy arrangements. If and when these payments are amended to include uncut pigs,

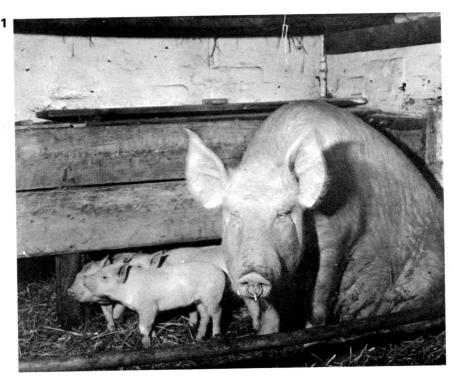
1

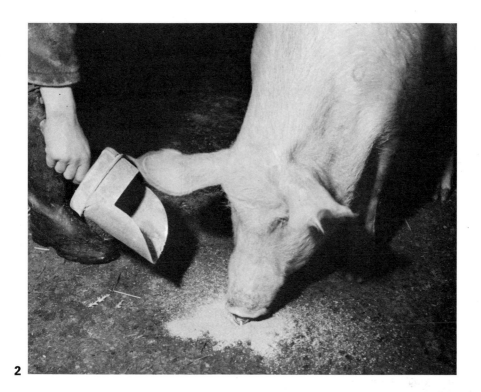

2

then the need for castration will be reduced to a minimum. In fact, with the continued improvements in pig husbandry, it may soon be possible to abolish pig castration altogether. The sooner the better so far as I'm concerned.

However, in the meantime, this unpleasant operation has to be done mostly by farmers and undoubtedly a sound aseptic routine technique can do much to avoid losses and reduce pain.

Age To Castrate
Best age for castration is *between 2 and 3 weeks (photo 1)*. By that time piglets are strong enough to withstand the shock and yet have not grown enough for the pain and stress to be grossly excessive. Nonetheless, the pain is considerable.

Management Of The Sow
This factor is most important and is the one most often disregarded by pig-keepers. The simplest way is to entice the sow out of the pen with food and feed her some distance away from the 'battle-field' (photo 2).

The sow need not be fed from a trough; she will clean the meal up from a concrete floor without any waste.

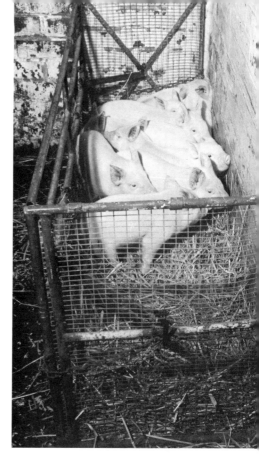

4

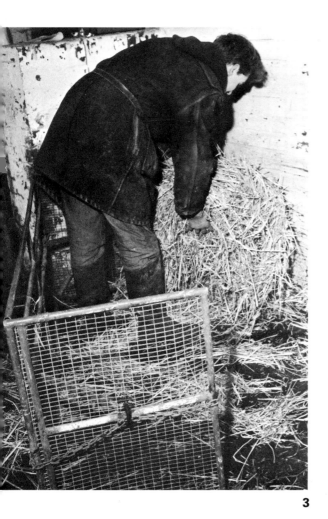

3

Cleanliness

It is essential that the piglets be kept on plenty of clean straw throughout the entire operation, so bed down one corner of the pen thickly *(photo 3)*.

Penning The Pigs

Probably the most difficult and certainly the most essential job is to keep the pigs on the straw in the corner. That is why every pig farmer should have a decent catching crate like this one *(photo 4)*. Improvisations with galvanised sheeting, old doors, etc., are most unsatisfactory as additional help is needed to hold the ends against the walls.

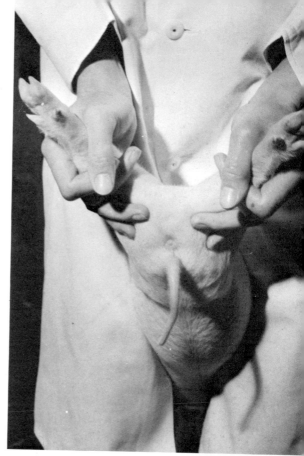

6

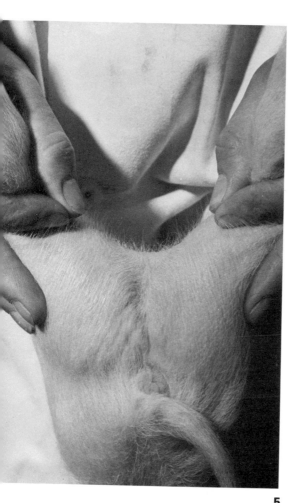

5

Best Way To Hold The Piglet

With the pig's shoulders held tightly between the knees the assistant should present its rear end to the operator *(photo 5)*.

During the demonstration my assistant had his fingers cut with the scalpel so I instructed him to hold the legs with the thumb and index finger only around the hock and the other fingers well out of the way. This is by far the better method of holding the pig *(photo 6)*.

Tools For The Job

Cotton-wool or gauze, antiseptic for the skin, antiseptic for the water, soap to

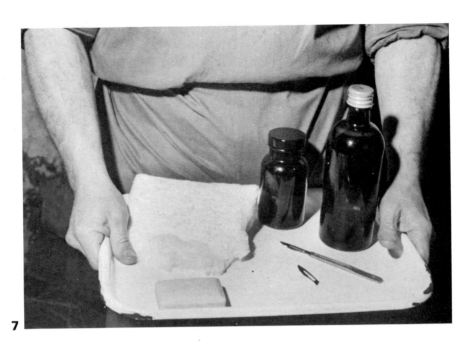

7

wash the hands and a scalpel with a spare blade *(photo 7)*. From the humane point of view it is essential that the blade should be razor sharp *(photo 8)*.

Hygiene

A bucket of hot water and a generous measure of a decent non-irritant antiseptic are essential *(photo 9)*.

8

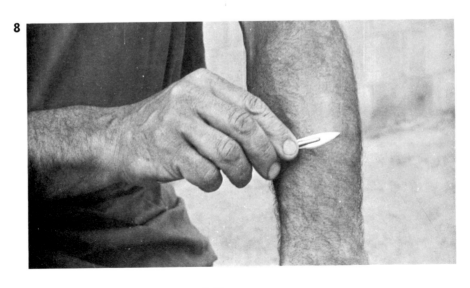

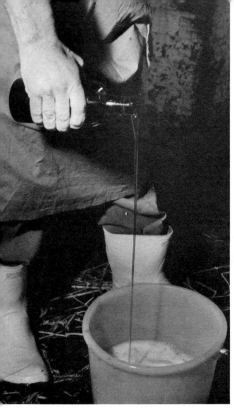

9

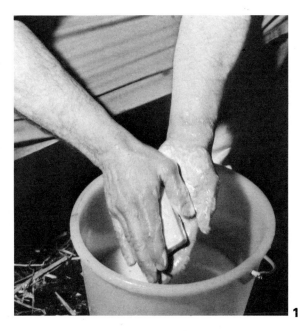

10

Scrub the hands thoroughly; if the wounds are going to become infected the operator's unclean hands are the most likely and dangerous source *(photo 10)*.

Another useful hint! After washing, dry the hands thoroughly on a clean towel or a piece of gauze *(photo 11)*. Wet slippery hands make the operation much more difficult.

11

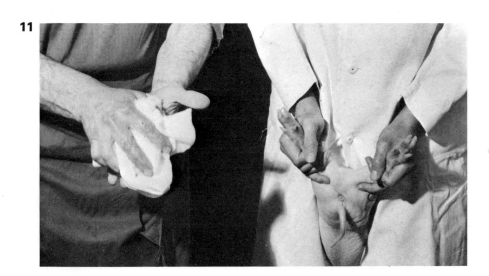

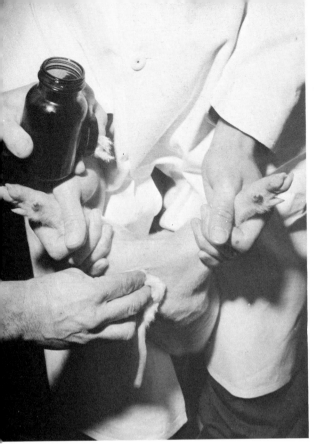

Before Cutting

Swab the entire area over with a reliable skin antiseptic *(photo 12)*. Your veterinary surgeon will be happy to prescribe one.

Getting The Testicle Up

First of all press the tips of the first and second fingers of the left hand (provided you are right-handed) into the groins of the piglet. This will bring the testicles into view *(photo 13)*.

Move the index finger away and slide the second finger into the groin on the side of the selected testicle *(photo 14)*.

12

13

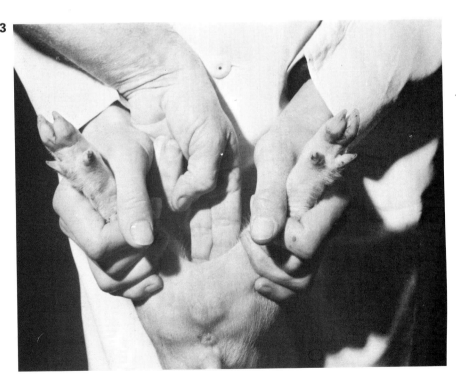

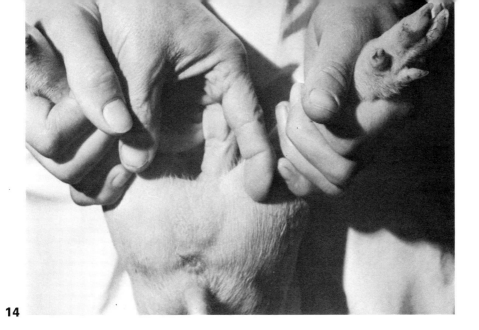

14

Still keeping the tip of the second finger firmly in the groin, bring the thumb and index finger to each side of the testicle and press inwards towards the second finger which is now pressing the testicle outwards *(photo 15)*.

Get the testicle hard against the skin so that the skin appears smooth and

15 ◗

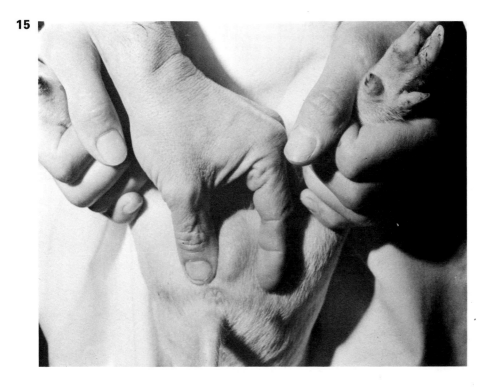

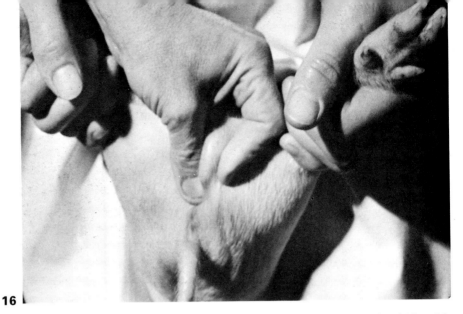

16

shiny *(photo 16)*. An old boss of mine used to tell me that you should be able to 'crack a nut' on the surface!

The Incision

The cut should be made at the base of the scrotum, i.e. at what will be the bottom of the testicle sac when the pig is standing up. This is done by starting the cut as close as possible to the palm or inner aspect of the index finger *(photo 17)*.

The cut needn't be any more than $\frac{1}{2}$ inch long. The obvious advantage of having the incision at the base of the scrotal sac is that it provides perfect

17

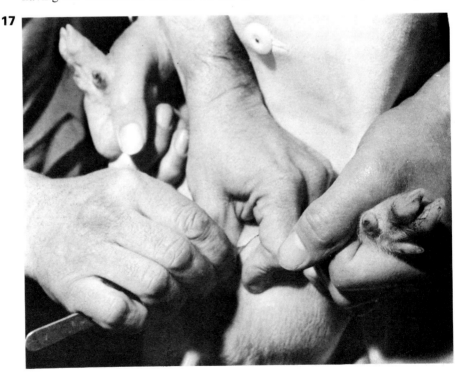

146

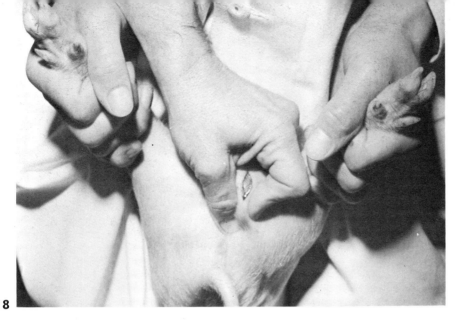

18

drainage, and prevents swelling and pocketing of infection *(photo 18)*.

What To Do Next

Another cut through the glistening membrane surrounding the testicle—and the testicle pops into view. It should be grasped between the thumb and palm of the left hand, and the index finger passed underneath the spermatic cord and pressed upwards. In this way the vascular (i.e. the parts containing the blood vessels) and non-vascular parts of the cord can be seen and differentiated *(photo 19)*.

19

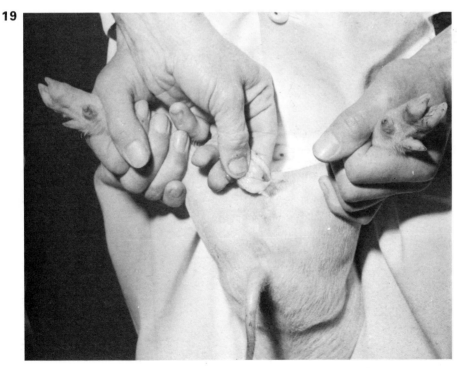

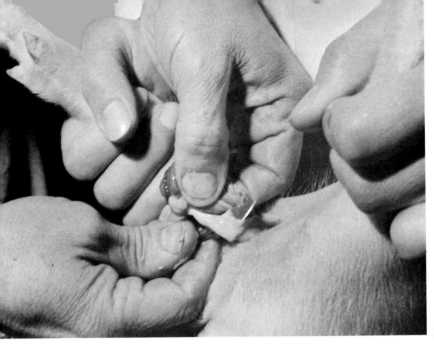

20

The scalpel is inserted between the red blood vessels and the white outer part of the cord; the cutting edge of the blade turned outwards; and the non-vascular part severed *(photo 20)*.

This leaves the vascular cord *(photo 21)* which can easily be identified by the red colour of the blood vessels.

21
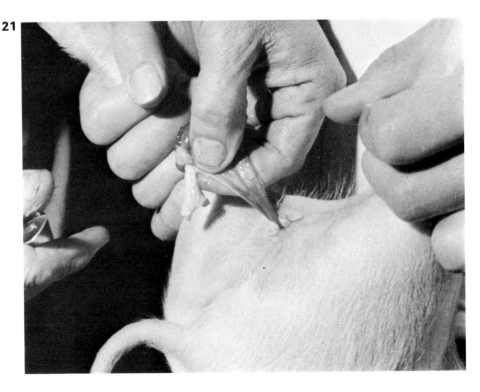

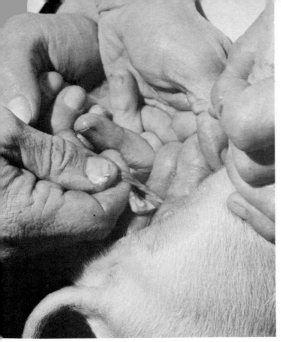 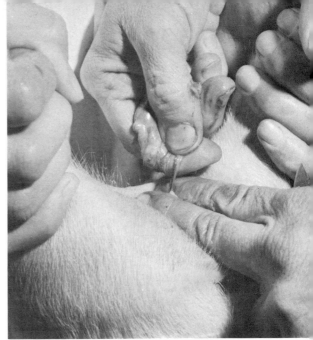

22   23

The testicle is now held in the right hand and the first and second fingers of the left hand pressed down firmly one on either side of the cord *(photo 22)*.

The testicle and cord are twisted once or twice around the right index finger *(photo 23)*.

The hands can be reversed according to the aptitude or preference of the operator *(photo 24)*.

24

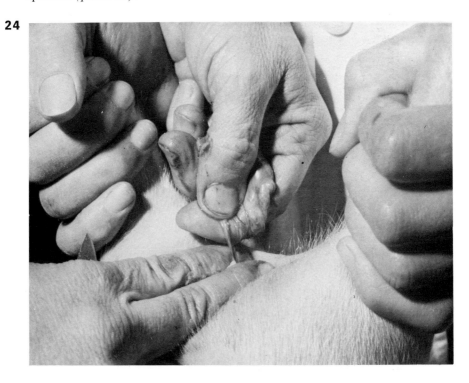

Last Stage Of The Operation

The vascular cord is 'stretched and drawn'; the abdominal part of the blood vessel then 'recoils' and the severed end 'turns inwards' thus preventing haemorrhage. If this technique is followed rigorously little or no bleeding will ever occur—even in larger pigs *(photo 25)*.

Final Precautions

A dust over with an antiseptic powder is a wise precaution against infection and always well worth while *(photo 26)*.

Lastly and very important—hold the piglet by the tail and return him into the bed of deep clean straw (photo 27). Mark him with a marking stick, but don't on any account let him run loose in the pen during the squeals of his fellow-sufferers. If you do you are asking for wound contamination and will certainly get it.

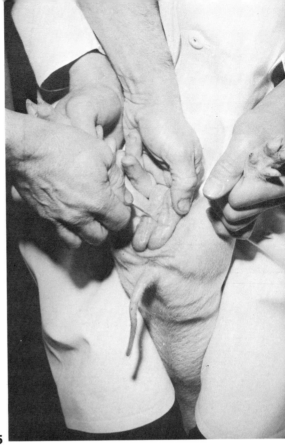

25

27 **26**

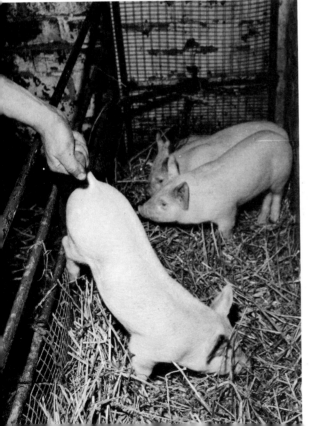

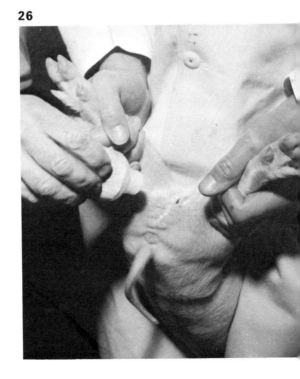

150

5
De-tusking

TRIMMING a boar's tusks, which should be a routine task, is a job the pig-man can do by himself. Too often it is neglected until a sow or attendant is attacked.

Tools For The Job

To cut a boar's tusks you require a strong, thin nylon rope, some 'embryotomy' wire (used by veterinary surgeons for cutting up calves inside cows), a roll of adhesive bandage and two pieces of wood *(photo 1)*. The wire (specially de-

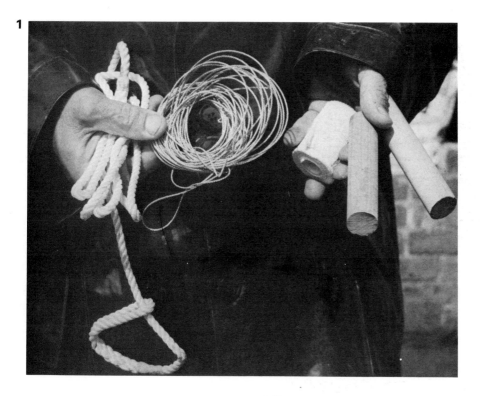

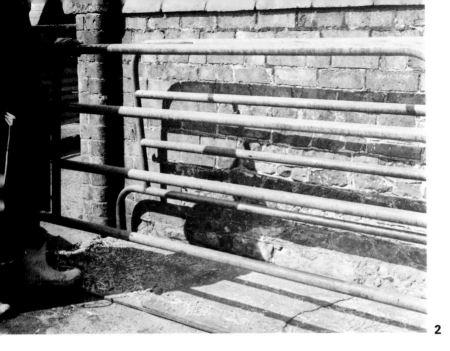

2

signed for 'sawing') can be obtained from your vet. To make the 'saw', cut a short length of the wire—about 3 feet long. Tie both ends around the centres of the wooden handles, and bind over the wire and knots on the handle with the adhesive bandage.

Place a strong metal crate at the entrance to a pen and sprinkle some food on the wooden floor of the crate *(photo 2)*.

3

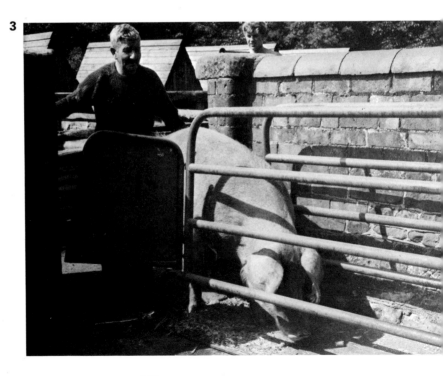

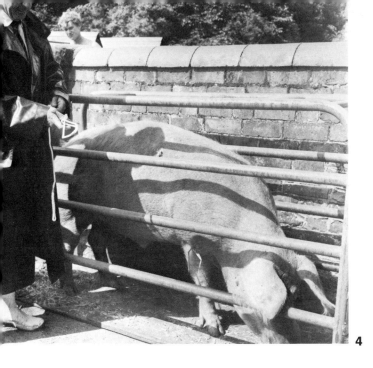

4

A metal farrowing crate is ideal—the boar will walk in quietly, eating the food as he goes *(photo 3)*.

When the boar is inside the crate and the rear door shut, take the thin nylon rope and make a running noose at one end *(photo 4)*.

Open the noose *(photo 5)* and drop it over the snout and upper jaw of the boar, working all the while from behind the head.

5

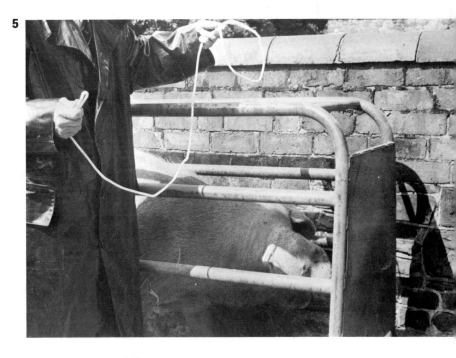

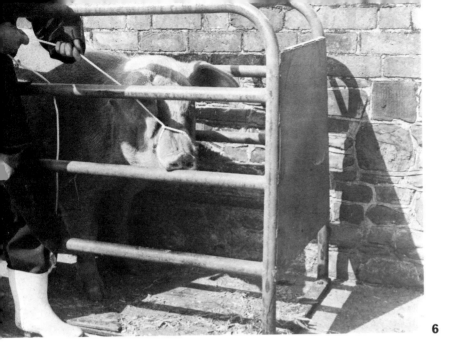

6

After the rope is in position, pull the noose tight *(photo 6)*.

Lift the boar's head as high as possible and wind the free end of the rope several times round the top bar of the crate *(photo 7)*. The boar's head is now in the correct position for the operation, with the offending tusks clearly exposed.

The bottom tusks are the dangerous ones because the points are constantly stropped and sharpened by contact with the upper tusks as the boar opens and shuts his mouth.

7
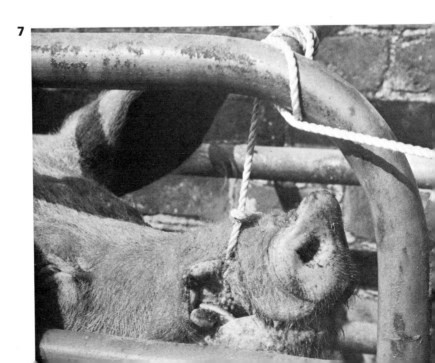

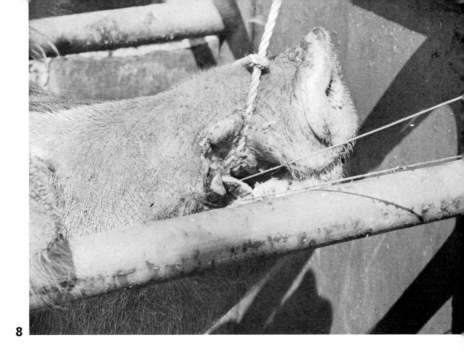

8

Slip the centre of the wire over the first lower tusk and pass the wire down to approximately $\frac{1}{8}$ inch above the gum *(photo 8)*. This is the correct depth to aim for: any lower will mean cutting the gum and possibly also the pulp cavity of the tooth, either of which would give the boar considerable pain.

Once the wire is fixed in position, saw leisurely through the tooth while keeping the wire in line with the gum *(photo 9)*.

Repeat the sawing with the upper tusk, this time keeping well clear of and parallel to the gum. It is not essential to take this tusk off as short as the lower

9

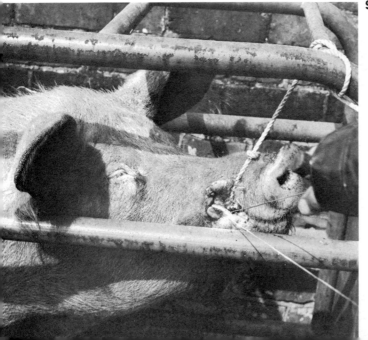

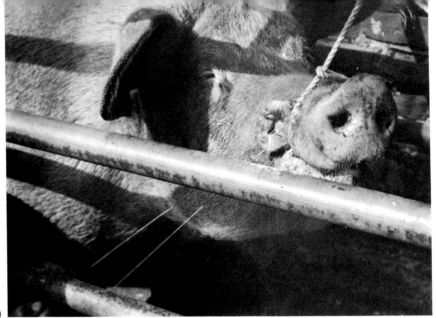

10

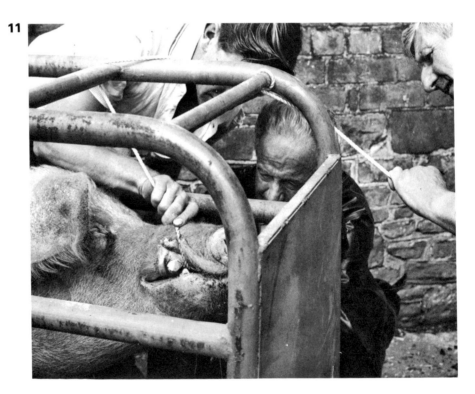

11

one because rarely, if ever, does it become dangerous. To keep parallel with the upper gum it is usually necessary to saw in a downward direction *(photo 10)*.

Refix the rope at the other side of the crate and repeat the sawing process with the opposite tusks *(photo 11)*.

The entire job should not take more than a quarter of an hour.

Index